Chair Yoga
For Women to Lose Weight

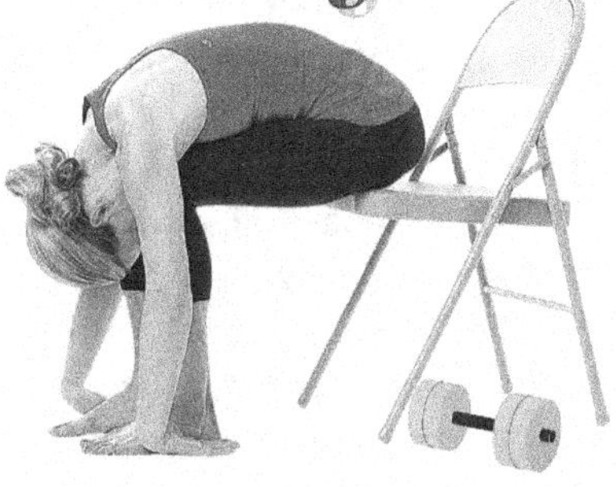

Exercise to Shed Belly Fat Enhance Mobility Flexibility and Strength with Intermediate Posture Poses

Forrest Vargas

For free consultation and assistance on Chair Yoga For Women to Lose Weight feel free to contact me with questions or for more information.
Forrestinstructor5@gmail.com

Strength is not just
about what you can
lift but also about
what you can
overcome

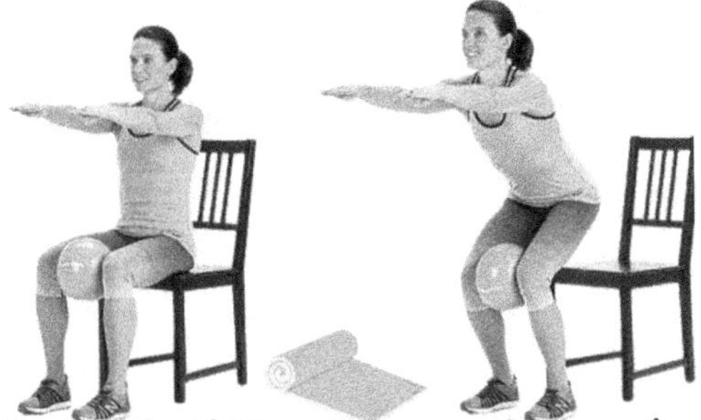

Flexibility is not just
bending your body
but bending your
mind to new
possibilities

ABOUT THE AUTHOR

Forrest Vargas, the author of "Chair Yoga for Women to Lose Weight," is a seasoned yoga instructor and wellness coach dedicated to empowering individuals to achieve holistic health and vitality. With over a decade of experience in the field, Forrest combines her expertise in yoga, fitness, and nutrition to offer a comprehensive approach to weight loss and wellness.

As a passionate advocate for accessible fitness, she specializes in Chair Yoga, making the practice inclusive and attainable for people of all ages and fitness levels. Her unique blend of gentle movements, mindful breathing, and targeted poses not only aids in weight loss but also improves mobility, flexibility, and strength.

Forrest's compassionate and encouraging teaching style, coupled with her deep understanding of the mind-body connection, inspires readers to embark on a transformative journey toward better health and self-discovery. Through her book, Forrest shares her wealth of knowledge and empowers women to embrace their inner strength, reclaim their health, and live their best lives.

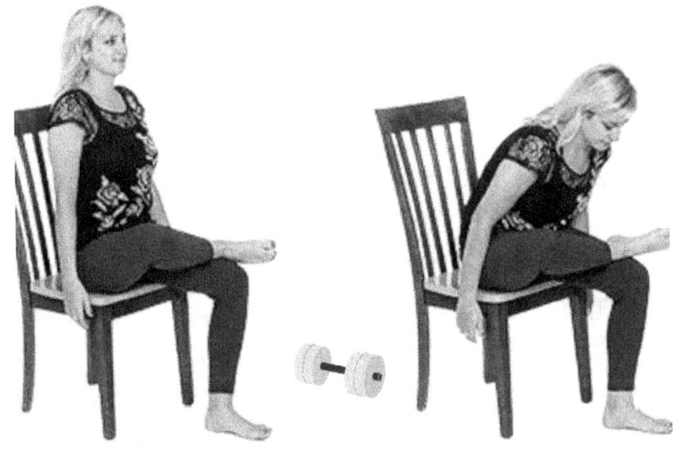

TABLE OF CONTENT

INTRODUCTION

In the hustle and bustle of modern life, it's all too easy to neglect our health and well-being. For Felicia, a busy working mother juggling multiple responsibilities, this reality hit home with a forceful urgency. Struggling with excess weight and feeling the strain of sedentary habits, Felicia longed for a solution that could seamlessly integrate into her hectic routine. Little did she know, her journey towards transformation would begin with a simple yet profound practice: Chair Yoga.

Felicia's story is not unique. Like many of us, she found herself caught in the whirlwind of daily obligations, neglecting her own needs in the process. But when she discovered Chair Yoga, everything changed. With the guidance of experienced instructor Forrest Vargas, Felicia embarked on a path of self-discovery and empowerment. Through gentle movements and mindful breathing, she not only shed unwanted pounds but also gained newfound vitality and confidence.

In this book, "Chair Yoga for Women to Lose Weight," Forrest Vargas shares Felicia's journey and invites you to embark on your own transformational path. Whether you're a busy professional, a stay-at-home parent, or anyone seeking a gentle yet effective way to improve your health, this book is your comprehensive guide. Through illustrated poses, expert tips, and practical advice, you'll discover how Chair Yoga can help you not only lose weight but also enhance mobility, flexibility, and strength. It's time to reclaim your health, reignite your inner spark, and embrace the transformative power of Chair Yoga.

CHAPTER 1

Overview of Chair Yoga

Chair Yoga offers a unique and accessible approach to physical fitness and well-being, making it an ideal practice for women seeking a gentle yet effective way to lose weight. This overview explores the foundational principles, benefits, and the transformative potential that Chair Yoga holds for women on their weight loss journey.

At its core, Chair Yoga adapts traditional yoga poses and principles to be performed while seated or supported by a chair. This modification opens the practice to a broader audience, making it particularly suitable for individuals with mobility challenges, beginners, or those who prefer a less strenuous approach to exercise. The emphasis on seated postures doesn't diminish the effectiveness but rather provides a gateway to holistic health for women of all ages and fitness levels.

One of the key attractions of Chair Yoga is its inclusivity. By eliminating the barrier of having to perform poses on the floor, it welcomes individuals who may find traditional yoga physically demanding or intimidating. This inclusivity extends its reach to those with limited mobility, joint issues, or anyone recovering from injuries, creating a more accessible avenue for women to embark on a fitness journey.

Outside of the physical world, chair yoga has many advantages.The practice incorporates breathwork and mindfulness, fostering a deep mind-body connection. This holistic approach is particularly beneficial for women looking to manage stress, improve mental well-being, and address emotional aspects linked to weight loss. Chair Yoga becomes a mindful journey that goes beyond shedding pounds; it becomes a transformative practice for overall health and balance.

The gentle nature of Chair Yoga doesn't compromise its efficacy in promoting weight loss. Seated postures engage core muscles, enhance flexibility, and contribute to the development of lean muscle mass. Additionally, the practice stimulates blood circulation, supporting metabolism and aiding in the burning of calories. As women embrace the poses and sequences, they find a sustainable and enjoyable way to incorporate physical activity into their daily lives, a crucial element in any weight loss endeavor.

Chair Yoga also serves as a gateway to improved posture and body awareness. Women often face challenges related to prolonged periods of sitting or sedentary lifestyles. Chair Yoga counteracts these issues by encouraging proper alignment and strengthening postural muscles. The emphasis on body awareness lays the foundation for mindful eating habits and lifestyle choices, creating a holistic approach to weight management.

Furthermore, the adaptability of Chair Yoga allows for personalized modifications, catering to individual needs and fitness levels. Instructors and practitioners can tailor sequences to address specific weight loss goals, making the practice versatile and accommodating for various health conditions or fitness objectives.

The overview of Chair Yoga wouldn't be complete without acknowledging its impact on stress reduction. Stress is a significant factor influencing weight gain, and Chair Yoga provides a sanctuary for women to unwind and release tension. Incorporating relaxation techniques and mindfulness into the practice establishes a harmonious balance between physical activity and mental well-being.

In essence, Chair Yoga for women seeking to lose weight offers a holistic and inclusive approach to wellness. It transcends the conventional notions of exercise, providing a gentle yet potent avenue for transformation. As women embrace the principles of Chair Yoga, they embark on a journey that not only shapes their physical bodies but also nurtures a profound connection between mind, body, and spirit. It is a journey towards sustainable weight loss that goes beyond the external and dives deep into the core of holistic well-being.

Benefits for Women and Weight Loss

The benefits of Chair Yoga for women extend far beyond the physical realm, encompassing mental, emotional, and holistic well-being. As a tailored approach to fitness, Chair Yoga offers a plethora of advantages that make it an ideal practice for those seeking to lose weight while fostering overall health.

1. Gentle and Accessible Fitness

Chair Yoga serves as a gateway to fitness, especially for women who may face physical limitations or are new to exercise. The practice's gentle nature allows individuals to engage in a meaningful fitness routine without the intimidation that can accompany more rigorous workouts. The use of a chair for support makes it accessible to women of all ages and fitness levels, providing a safe and inclusive space for physical activity.

2. Adaptable for Varied Fitness Levels

One of the standout benefits of Chair Yoga is its adaptability. Whether a woman is a beginner, dealing with mobility challenges, or recovering from an injury, the practice can be modified to suit her specific needs. Instructors can customize poses and sequences, ensuring that participants can progress at their own pace. This adaptability promotes a sense of accomplishment and empowerment, crucial factors in sustaining motivation for weight loss.

3.Effective for Core Strength and Toning

Contrary to the misconception that seated exercises may not be as effective, Chair Yoga engages core muscles in a meaningful way. Seated postures and targeted movements work to strengthen the abdominal muscles and promote overall core stability. This engagement not only contributes to toning but also lays the foundation for improved posture, a key element in both physical aesthetics and long-term weight management.

4. Flexibility Enhancement

Chair Yoga incorporates a variety of stretches that enhance flexibility, targeting different muscle groups. Improved flexibility is not only essential for the prevention of injuries but also contributes to a sense of vitality and well-being. As women gradually embrace the practice, they find increased ease of movement, promoting an active lifestyle that complements weight loss efforts.

5.Mind-Body Connection and Emotional Well-Being

Beyond the physical benefits, Chair Yoga places a strong emphasis on the mind-body connection. The integration of breathwork and mindfulness creates a holistic approach to wellness. Women engaging in Chair Yoga often report reduced stress levels, improved mood, and a heightened sense of self-awareness.Establishing a solid foundation for long-term weight loss requires managing emotional eating and other associated factors.

6.Metabolism Boost and Calorie Burning

Chair Yoga, despite its gentleness, stimulates blood circulation and supports metabolism. The combination of seated poses, controlled movements, and conscious breathing contributes to calorie burning. While it may not be as high-intensity as some other forms of exercise, Chair Yoga offers a sustainable and enjoyable way to incorporate physical activity into daily life, aiding in weight loss over time.

7. Posture Improvement

Many women face challenges related to poor posture due to sedentary lifestyles or extended periods of sitting. Chair Yoga addresses this issue by encouraging proper alignment and strengthening postural muscles. Improved posture not only enhances physical appearance but also plays a crucial role in promoting overall body awareness, influencing positive lifestyle choices related to weight management.

8.Stress Reduction and Emotional Eating Management

Stress is a significant factor influencing weight gain, particularly for women. Chair Yoga provides a sanctuary for relaxation, incorporating techniques to manage stress effectively. As stress levels decrease, women are better equipped to make mindful choices about their diet and lifestyle. This emotional resilience is a valuable asset in the journey towards sustainable weight loss.

9.Personal Empowerment and Confidence Building

The adaptability and inclusivity of Chair Yoga contribute to a sense of personal empowerment. As women see progress in their flexibility, strength, and overall well-being, it boosts confidence and self-esteem. This positive self-image becomes a powerful motivator in adhering to a weight loss journey, fostering a sustainable commitment to healthier choices.

10. Holistic Wellness Journey

Chair Yoga goes beyond being a mere exercise routine; it becomes a holistic wellness journey. Women engaging in the practice not only witness physical transformations but also experience a profound shift in their overall approach to health. It becomes a lifestyle choice that encompasses mindful movement, stress management, and a balanced perspective on weight loss.

The benefits of Chair Yoga for women on the path to weight loss are multifaceted. From physical fitness to emotional well-being, the practice offers a comprehensive and sustainable approach. As women embrace Chair Yoga, they discover not only the joy of movement but also a transformative journey towards holistic wellness. It becomes a mindful and empowering practice, weaving its positive impact into various facets of their lives.

CHAPTER 2

Getting Started with Chair Yoga

"Getting Started with Chair Yoga" is the foundational step on the transformative journey towards holistic well-being for women of all ages and fitness levels. This section serves as a guide to creating a comfortable and inclusive space for the practice, choosing the right chair, and understanding essential safety precautions.

1. Creating a Comfortable Space

Before diving into Chair Yoga, it's crucial to establish a dedicated and comfortable space for practice. This area should be free from distractions, providing a serene environment that encourages focus and relaxation. Consider incorporating elements like soft lighting, calming colors, and perhaps soothing background music to enhance the overall experience. The goal is to create a space that invites women to connect with themselves, fostering a sense of tranquility and mindfulness during their Chair Yoga sessions.

2. Choosing the Right Chair

The choice of chair plays a pivotal role in the effectiveness of Chair Yoga. Opt for a sturdy and stable chair without arms, allowing for a full range of movement. The seat should be flat and level to ensure proper alignment during seated poses. Additionally, the chair's height should allow the feet to rest comfortably on the floor. By selecting an appropriate chair, women can engage in Chair Yoga with confidence, knowing that their practice is supported by a stable foundation.

3. Understanding Safety Precautions

Safety is paramount in any fitness routine, and Chair Yoga is no exception. This section outlines essential safety precautions to ensure a risk-free and enjoyable experience. Participants are encouraged to listen to their bodies, avoiding any movements that cause pain or discomfort. Clear instructions on proper posture and alignment are provided, emphasizing the importance of maintaining a balance between challenge and ease. Additionally, individuals with specific health concerns or pre-existing conditions are advised to consult with a healthcare professional before embarking on their Chair Yoga journey.

4. Gentle Warm-Up Exercises

To prepare the body for the practice ahead, "Getting Started with Chair Yoga" introduces gentle warm-up exercises. These movements focus on loosening up the joints, improving circulation, and awakening the muscles. Warm-up exercises serve as a bridge between stillness and movement, gradually transitioning women into the dynamic and mindful nature of Chair Yoga. Proper warm-up sets the tone for a more fluid and enjoyable practice, reducing the risk of injury and ensuring optimal engagement.

5.Breathwork Techniques for Relaxation

Incorporating breathwork is a fundamental aspect of "Getting Started with Chair Yoga." This section introduces women to the transformative power of conscious breathing. Simple yet effective techniques, such as deep diaphragmatic breathing and rhythmic breath awareness, are explored. Breathwork not only enhances oxygenation of the body but also promotes relaxation, reducing stress and preparing the mind for the meditative aspects of Chair Yoga. By mastering breath control, women can cultivate a deeper connection between their breath and movement, enriching their overall yoga experience.

6. Seated Postures for Beginners

Building a strong foundation is essential for the success of any yoga practice. "Getting Started with Chair Yoga" introduces basic seated postures tailored for beginners. These poses focus on cultivating awareness of body alignment, encouraging gentle stretches, and laying the groundwork for more advanced postures. Emphasis is placed on maintaining proper form and listening to the body's cues, empowering women to gradually progress in their practice with confidence and ease.

In essence, "Getting Started with Chair Yoga" is the gateway to a transformative journey. It establishes the groundwork for a safe, inclusive, and enjoyable practice. By creating a comfortable space, choosing the right chair, understanding safety precautions, incorporating gentle warm-up exercises, and embracing breathwork and beginner-friendly seated postures, women are equipped with the tools and knowledge to embark on a holistic and empowering Chair Yoga experience.

Choosing the Right Chair

Selecting the right chair is a pivotal step in ensuring a comfortable and effective Chair Yoga practice. The choice of chair significantly influences the quality of the experience, impacting stability, range of motion, and overall support during the practice. This section delves into the key considerations for choosing an appropriate chair and provides guidance to empower women in making informed decisions for their Chair Yoga journey.

1. Stability and Sturdiness

The first and foremost consideration when choosing a chair for Chair Yoga is its stability and sturdiness. Opt for a chair with a solid frame and a broad, stable base. The chair should withstand the shifts in weight and movement associated with yoga poses, providing a secure foundation for practitioners. Stability is crucial for instilling confidence, allowing women to focus on the practice without concerns about the chair's integrity.

2. Armless Design for Freedom of Movement

An optimal Chair Yoga chair design features no arms. This armless structure ensures unobstructed movement and allows for a full range of motion during seated poses and stretches. The absence of arms permits the arms to move freely, facilitating fluid transitions between postures. This design choice contributes to the accessibility of the practice, accommodating various body shapes and sizes.

3. Appropriate Seat Height

The chair's seat height is a critical factor in maintaining proper alignment during Chair Yoga. Ideally, the feet should rest flat on the floor with knees bent at a comfortable angle. This configuration ensures a stable foundation and allows for proper engagement of leg muscles. Chairs with adjustable heights offer versatility, allowing practitioners to tailor the chair to their individual needs and preferences.

4. Flat and Level Seat Surface

The seat surface of the chair should be flat and level to support correct alignment of the spine and pelvis. A level seat prevents practitioners from tilting forward or backward during poses, promoting a neutral and stable posture. This feature is essential for the effectiveness of seated postures and contributes to the overall comfort of the practice.

5. Comfortable Yet Firm Cushioning

While comfort is key, the chair's cushioning should strike a balance between comfort and firmness. Too much softness may hinder stability and proper alignment, while too much firmness may lead to discomfort during prolonged sessions. Opt for a chair with supportive yet comfortable cushioning, ensuring a pleasant experience without compromising the structural integrity needed for Chair Yoga poses.

6. Non-Slip Base

To prevent unintended movement during the practice, the chair should have a non-slip base. This feature enhances safety by minimizing the risk of the chair sliding on smooth surfaces. A non-slip base provides practitioners with the assurance that the chair will remain securely in place, allowing them to focus on the mindful movements and poses without distraction.

7. Easy to Clean and Maintain

Practicality is another aspect to consider when choosing a Chair Yoga chair.Choose a chair that requires little upkeep and is easy to clean.This is especially relevant if the chair is used in various settings or shared among multiple practitioners. A chair with a durable and easy-to-clean material ensures hygiene and longevity, making it a practical investment for long-term use.

By carefully considering these factors, women can select a chair that aligns with their individual needs, enhancing the overall experience of Chair Yoga. The right chair becomes not just a supportive prop but an integral partner in the journey towards improved flexibility, strength, and holistic well-being. As women embark on their Chair Yoga practice with a thoughtfully chosen chair, they set the stage for a transformative and empowering wellness journey.

Creating a Comfortable Space

Creating a comfortable space is an essential element in establishing an inviting and conducive environment for Chair Yoga practice. This dedicated space becomes a sanctuary where women can immerse themselves in the mindful movements, breathwork, and relaxation inherent in Chair Yoga. This section explores the key components of crafting a comfortable space that enhances the overall experience and encourages a deeper connection with the practice.

1. Mindful Design and Ambiance

Begin by considering the design and ambiance of the space. Opt for a room or corner with ample natural light, if possible, to create a bright and uplifting atmosphere. Select calming colors for the walls or incorporate soft furnishings that evoke a sense of tranquility. The intention is to create a space that encourages mindfulness and relaxation, setting the stage for a positive and immersive Chair Yoga experience.

2. Declutter and Simplify

A clutter-free environment promotes focus and concentration during Chair Yoga practice. Clear the space of unnecessary items, allowing for an unobstructed flow of movement. Keep only the essential props and accessories, such as the chair, yoga mat, and any additional supportive tools. Simplifying the space minimizes distractions, fostering a serene backdrop that enhances the mind-body connection.

3. Personal Touch and Inspiration

Infuse the space with personal touches and elements that inspire. Consider adding items like plants, candles, or artwork that hold personal significance or evoke a sense of calm. These elements contribute to a sense of ownership over the space, making it more inviting and encouraging women to return to their practice regularly.

4. Comfortable Flooring

While Chair Yoga primarily involves seated and supported poses, having a comfortable flooring option can enhance the overall experience. Consider placing a yoga mat or a soft rug under the chair. This provides a cushioned surface for seated postures and adds a touch of comfort to the space. The flooring should complement the overall design while prioritizing practicality and comfort.

5. Adequate Ventilation

Ensuring proper ventilation is essential for creating a comfortable space. Adequate airflow contributes to a fresh and invigorating atmosphere, preventing the space from feeling stagnant during practice. Open windows, use a fan, or incorporate natural air purifiers like plants to maintain a well-ventilated environment that supports a sense of vitality and well-being.

6. Proper Lighting

Appropriate lighting plays a crucial role in enhancing the ambiance of the space. Ideally, incorporate adjustable lighting options to cater to different preferences and times of day. Soft, warm lighting can create a cozy atmosphere for evening sessions, while bright, natural light is beneficial for daytime practice. Lighting that can be adjusted allows women to customize the space based on their mood and preferences.

7. Distraction-Free Zone

Encourage practitioners to designate their Chair Yoga space as a distraction-free zone. Silence phones, close doors, and communicate to others in the household about the dedicated practice time. Minimizing external disturbances allows women to fully immerse themselves in the present moment, fostering a deeper connection with their breath, movement, and the overall experience of Chair Yoga.

8. Temperature Control

Maintaining a comfortable temperature is crucial for an enjoyable practice.Make sure the temperature in the room is just right—neither hot nor cold. Consider the use of blankets or layers that can be easily adjusted to accommodate individual comfort levels. A moderate and consistent temperature contributes to a comfortable environment, supporting relaxation and ease of movement during Chair Yoga.

9. Soundscapes and Music

Integrating soothing sounds or music into the space can enhance the overall experience of Chair Yoga. Consider creating playlists with calming instrumental music or nature sounds. The auditory backdrop adds an additional layer of relaxation, creating a multisensory environment that elevates the practice to a holistic and immersive level.

By paying attention to these aspects, women can curate a space that nurtures their Chair Yoga practice. This thoughtfully crafted environment becomes a personal retreat, encouraging a sense of mindfulness, relaxation, and connection with the transformative journey of Chair Yoga for women on their path to improved well-being and weight loss.

Safety Precautions

Ensuring safety during Chair Yoga is paramount to provide participants with a secure and comfortable environment for their practice. This section outlines essential safety precautions that women should be mindful of as they embark on their Chair Yoga journey. These precautions serve as guidelines to promote a positive and injury-free experience, emphasizing the importance of listening to one's body and practicing within individual comfort levels.

1. Listen to Your Body

One of the fundamental safety precautions in Chair Yoga is the encouragement to listen to one's body. Participants should be attuned to how their body responds to each movement and pose. If a particular posture causes discomfort or pain, it is essential to modify or skip that pose. This mindful approach helps prevent strain and minimizes the risk of injuries during the practice.

2. Gentle Warm-Up and Cool Down

Commencing the Chair Yoga session with a gentle warm-up is crucial to prepare the body for movement. Warm-up exercises help increase blood circulation, improve flexibility, and reduce the risk of injury. Similarly, incorporating a cool-down segment at the end of the practice aids in bringing the heart rate back to normal and promoting a sense of relaxation.

3. Proper Posture and Alignment

Emphasizing proper posture and alignment is a key safety consideration. Participants should be guided on maintaining correct body alignment during seated poses to prevent unnecessary strain on the spine, shoulders, and neck. Educating women on the importance of maintaining a neutral spine and proper alignment fosters a safe and effective Chair Yoga practice.

4. Be Mindful of Joint Health

Many Chair Yoga poses involve joint movement, and it's crucial to be mindful of individual joint health. Participants with specific joint concerns or conditions should approach movements with caution, opting for modifications when needed. Supporting joint health ensures a sustainable and injury-free practice over the long term.

5. Adapt Poses to Individual Ability

Chair Yoga is inherently adaptable, allowing for modifications based on individual abilities. Safety lies in tailoring poses to suit each participant's comfort level and physical condition. Instructors should encourage participants to embrace variations and use props as needed to ensure a practice that is both safe and fulfilling.

6. Avoid Overexertion

While Chair Yoga is a gentle practice, participants should be cautious not to overexert themselves. Pushing beyond one's limits may lead to fatigue, muscle strain, or potential injury. The practice is designed to be accessible and enjoyable, promoting gradual progress rather than aggressive exertion.

7. Communicate with Instructors

Effective communication with Chair Yoga instructors is a crucial safety measure. Participants are encouraged to share any health concerns, limitations, or recent injuries before the session begins. This information allows instructors to tailor the practice, provide appropriate modifications, and ensure a safe experience for everyone involved.

8. Stay Hydrated

Maintaining proper hydration is a general safety consideration for any physical activity. Encourage participants to have water nearby and take sips as needed during the session. Staying hydrated supports overall well-being and helps prevent dehydration-related issues.

9. Use Supportive Props

The incorporation of supportive props, such as cushions or blocks, can enhance stability and comfort during Chair Yoga. Participants should be guided on how to use these props effectively to modify poses and provide additional support when necessary. Using props appropriately contributes to a safer and more enjoyable practice.

By incorporating these safety precautions into their Chair Yoga practice, women can cultivate an environment that prioritizes well-being and minimizes the risk of injuries. The emphasis on mindfulness, proper alignment, and individual adaptation creates a foundation for a positive and sustainable Chair Yoga experience on the journey toward improved health and weight loss.

CHAPTER 3

The Basics of Chair Yoga Poses

"The Basics of Chair Yoga Poses" serves as a fundamental guide for women embarking on their Chair Yoga journey. This section introduces foundational seated postures, gentle warm-up exercises, and essential breathwork techniques. These basic elements lay the groundwork for a safe, accessible, and enjoyable Chair Yoga practice, emphasizing the integration of movement, breath, and mindfulness.

1. Gentle Warm-Up Exercises

The journey into Chair Yoga begins with gentle warm-up exercises designed to prepare the body for movement. These may include seated neck stretches, shoulder rolls, and wrist rotations. The aim is to awaken muscles, improve blood circulation, and create a sense of physical readiness for the upcoming poses. Warm-up exercises serve as a bridge between stillness and movement, easing participants into the mindful flow of Chair Yoga.

2. Seated Mountain Pose (Tadasana)

This foundational pose establishes the principles of proper alignment and posture. Participants sit tall on the chair, grounding through the feet, engaging the core, and reaching the arms overhead. Seated Mountain Pose promotes spinal awareness, strengthens the core, and sets the tone for mindful seated postures.

3.Seated Forward Bend (Paschimottanasana)

A gentle forward bend allows participants to stretch the spine and hamstrings while seated on the chair. Leaning forward from the hips with a straight back, women experience a gentle release in the lower back and increased flexibility in the hamstrings. The focus on controlled movement and breath creates a meditative quality to the pose.

4.Seated Twist (Ardha Matsyendrasana)

Seated twists help improve spinal mobility and promote digestion. Participants gently rotate their torso, using the backrest of the chair for support. The twist engages the core and encourages a sense of detoxification and release. Controlled breathing complements the twist, enhancing the overall therapeutic benefits of the pose.

5. Seated Cat-Cow Stretch

Adapting the traditional Cat-Cow Stretch to a seated position on the chair brings fluidity to the spine. Participants alternate between arching and rounding the back, syncing the movement with breath. Seated Cat-Cow Stretch fosters spinal flexibility, releases tension in the back, and promotes a sense of dynamic movement within the seated practice.

6. Chest Opener

The Chest Opener pose involves sitting at the edge of the chair, opening the arms wide, and gently squeezing the shoulder blades together. This pose counters the effects of prolonged sitting, encourages good posture, and provides a stretch across the chest and shoulders. The expansion of the chest promotes deep breathing and a sense of openness.

7. Seated Warrior (Virabhadrasana)

Adapting the Warrior pose to a seated variation on the chair brings strength and stability. Participants engage their core and reach their arms overhead, creating a lengthening effect through the spine. Seated Warrior fosters strength in the upper body and core muscles while encouraging participants to feel grounded and empowered.

8. Breathwork Techniques

Introducing breathwork is an integral part of the basics of Chair Yoga. Techniques such as diaphragmatic breathing, where participants focus on deep inhalations and exhalations, promote relaxation and mindfulness. Integrating breath awareness into each pose enhances the mind-body connection and cultivates a sense of calm within the practice.

9. Seated Knee Hug

This gentle knee-to-chest pose provides a release for the lower back and hips. Participants bring one knee at a time towards the chest, hugging it gently. The pose encourages a connection with the breath and a release of tension in the lower back, fostering a sense of nurturing self-care.

10. Seated Relaxation (Savasana)

Every Chair Yoga session concludes with a seated relaxation pose. Participants sit comfortably, close their eyes, and focus on their breath. Seated Savasana allows for integration of the benefits from the practice, promoting a sense of calm and rejuvenation.

By incorporating these foundational Chair Yoga poses into their practice, women lay the groundwork for a holistic and mindful journey. The basics serve as a stepping stone towards more advanced postures, fostering increased flexibility, strength, and overall well-being on the path to weight loss and improved health.

Gentle Warm-Up Exercises

Gentle warm-up exercises are the essential prelude to a Chair Yoga session, serving to prepare the body, mind, and breath for the subsequent practice. These exercises are designed to increase blood flow, improve flexibility, and create a sense of physical and mental readiness. As participants engage in these gentle movements, they establish a connection with their bodies, fostering a mindful and soothing introduction to the Chair Yoga experience.

1. Neck Stretches

Initiating the warm-up with gentle neck stretches helps release tension and promote flexibility in the cervical spine. Participants perform slow and controlled neck rotations, moving the head from side to side and gently tilting it forward and backward. These movements enhance mobility, alleviate stiffness, and set the foundation for a relaxed and supple neck throughout the practice.

2. Shoulder Rolls

Seated shoulder rolls are an effective way to loosen up the upper body. Participants roll their shoulders forward and backward in a smooth and circular motion. This exercise helps release tension in the shoulders, neck, and upper back, promoting increased circulation and preparing the upper body for the range of movements in Chair Yoga poses.

3. Wrist Circles

Wrist circles are introduced to address the often-overlooked wrists, especially important for individuals who spend extended periods typing or engaged in repetitive hand movements. Participants gently rotate their wrists clockwise and then counterclockwise, promoting flexibility and relieving any stiffness in the wrist joints.

4. Ankle Flex and Point

Seated ankle flex and point exercises encourage mobility in the ankles and promote circulation in the lower limbs. Participants lift their feet slightly off the ground, alternating between flexing and pointing their toes. This gentle movement warms up the lower extremities, preparing them for the weight-bearing aspects of some Chair Yoga poses.

5. Seated Cat-Cow Stretch

Adapting the traditional Cat-Cow Stretch from mat-based yoga to a seated position on the chair brings a dynamic element to the warm-up. Participants arch and round their backs while seated, synchronizing the movement with their breath. This exercise encourages spinal flexibility, warms up the back muscles, and establishes a connection between breath and movement.

6. Seated Forward and Side Bends

Seated forward bends and side bends gently stretch the spine and sides of the torso. Participants reach forward, aiming to touch their toes or shins, and then lean gently to each side. These movements promote flexibility in the spine, engage the core muscles, and set the stage for seated yoga poses that involve lateral movements.

7. Seated Knee Lifts

Seated knee lifts engage the core and warm up the abdominal muscles. Participants lift one knee at a time towards the chest, alternating between legs. This exercise encourages abdominal awareness, enhances circulation, and provides a gentle activation of the core muscles in preparation for more dynamic Chair Yoga poses.

8. Seated Twist Preparations

Seated twist preparations involve gently rotating the torso from side to side while keeping the hips grounded. Participants can use the backrest of the chair for support. These twists promote spinal flexibility, engage the obliques, and prepare the spine for more advanced seated twists during the main Chair Yoga practice.

9. Diaphragmatic Breathing

Incorporating diaphragmatic breathing into the warm-up phase establishes a mindful connection between breath and movement. Participants focus on deep inhalations through the nose, allowing the diaphragm to expand fully, and exhale slowly through pursed lips. This intentional breathing calms the nervous system, prepares the body for the practice, and fosters a sense of presence.

10. Seated Gentle Shakeout

To conclude the warm-up, a seated shakeout helps release any remaining tension and energize the body. Participants gently shake their hands, arms, and legs while seated, allowing any residual stiffness to dissipate. This exercise brings a sense of vibrancy and prepares participants for the flowing movements and poses ahead in the Chair Yoga session.

In essence, these gentle warm-up exercises set the tone for a mindful and safe Chair Yoga practice. They provide a comprehensive preparation for the body, promoting flexibility, circulation, and a heightened awareness of breath and movement. As participants progress through these warm-up activities, they lay the groundwork for a positive and rejuvenating Chair Yoga experience.

Seated Postures for Beginners

Seated postures form the foundation of Chair Yoga, offering a gentle and accessible introduction for beginners. These poses focus on promoting flexibility, improving posture, and cultivating mindfulness. The beauty of seated postures is their adaptability, making them suitable for individuals of all ages and fitness levels. As beginners engage in these foundational poses, they initiate a journey into the transformative world of Chair Yoga, building strength and fostering a deeper mind-body connection.

1. Seated Mountain Pose (Tadasana)

Begin with the fundamental Seated Mountain Pose. Participants sit tall on the chair, grounding through the feet, and extending the arms overhead. This pose establishes proper alignment, promotes awareness of the breath, and creates a sense of rootedness.

2.Seated Forward Bend (Paschimottanasana)

Seated Forward Bend provides a gentle stretch for the spine and hamstrings. Participants hinge at the hips, reaching forward towards their toes or shins. This pose fosters flexibility in the lower back and hamstrings while encouraging a sense of surrender and release.

3.Seated Twist (Ardha Matsyendrasana)

Introduce the Seated Twist to enhance spinal mobility. Participants rotate their torso, using the chair's backrest for support. Seated Twist promotes a gentle detoxification, engages the core, and encourages a sense of revitalization.

4. Seated Side Stretch

Seated Side Stretch offers a simple yet effective way to release tension in the sides of the torso. Participants reach one arm overhead, gently leaning to the opposite side. This pose improves lateral flexibility and brings awareness to the breath and ribcage expansion.

5.Seated Butterfly Pose (Baddha Konasana)

Seated Butterfly Pose provides a gentle hip opener. Participants bring the soles of their feet together and allow their knees to drop outward. This pose encourages flexibility in the hips and inner thighs while promoting a sense of relaxation.

6. Seated Cat-Cow Stretch

Adapted from traditional yoga, Seated Cat-Cow Stretch brings fluidity to the spine. Participants alternate between arching and rounding their backs, syncing the movement with breath. This seated variation enhances spinal flexibility and introduces the concept of dynamic movement within a seated practice.

7. Seated Knee Hug

Seated Knee Hug offers a nurturing stretch for the lower back and hips. Participants bring one knee at a time towards the chest, gently hugging it. This pose provides a sense of comfort and encourages participants to connect with their breath while releasing tension.

8. Seated Warrior (Virabhadrasana)

Seated Warrior adapts the traditional Warrior pose to a seated variation. Participants engage their core and lift their arms overhead, creating a lengthening effect through the spine. Seated Warrior promotes strength in the upper body and a grounded sense of stability.

9.Seated Ankle-to-Knee Pose (Agnistambhasana)

Seated Ankle-to-Knee Pose offers a gentle stretch for the outer hips. Participants cross one ankle over the opposite knee, maintaining an upright posture. This pose encourages hip flexibility and awareness, fostering a sense of balance and ease.

10. Seated Relaxation (Savasana)

Conclude the sequence with Seated Relaxation, a moment for participants to sit comfortably, close their eyes, and focus on their breath. This seated variation of Savasana allows for integration of the benefits from the practice, promoting a sense of calm and rejuvenation.

As beginners explore these seated postures, they lay the groundwork for a fulfilling Chair Yoga practice. These foundational poses introduce key elements of flexibility, strength, and mindfulness, setting the stage for a journey of holistic well-being and exploration of deeper aspects of Chair Yoga.

Breathing Techniques for Relaxation

In Chair Yoga, incorporating specific breathing techniques is integral to promoting relaxation, reducing stress, and fostering a deeper mind-body connection. These techniques, often referred to as pranayama, guide participants to harness the power of their breath for greater tranquility and overall well-being. As individuals engage in these breathing practices, they cultivate a heightened sense of mindfulness and relaxation within the context of their seated practice.

1.Diaphragmatic Breathing (Abdominal or Belly Breathing)

Begin with Diaphragmatic Breathing, emphasizing deep inhalations and exhalations. Participants place one hand on the chest and the other on the abdomen. Inhale deeply through the nose, allowing the abdomen to expand fully. Exhale slowly through pursed lips, feeling the abdomen contract. This technique encourages relaxation, activates the diaphragm, and enhances oxygenation.

2.Three-Part Breath (Dirga Pranayama)

Introduce the Three-Part Breath to enhance lung capacity and deepen the breath. Inhale slowly through the nose, filling the lower, middle, and upper lungs sequentially. Exhale gradually, releasing the breath from the upper, middle, and lower lungs. This technique promotes a sense of balance and encourages a full, conscious breath cycle.

3. Ujjayi Breath (Victorious Breath)

Ujjayi Breath involves creating a subtle constriction in the back of the throat during both inhalation and exhalation. This technique results in a soft, audible sound resembling ocean waves. Ujjayi Breath promotes a focused and calming effect, guiding participants to synchronize breath with movement and fostering a meditative state.

4. Alternate Nostril Breathing (Nadi Shodhana)

Guide participants through Alternate Nostril Breathing to balance energy and promote relaxation. With the right thumb closing the right nostril and the ring finger closing the left nostril, participants inhale through one nostril and exhale through the other, alternating between sides. This technique encourages a sense of balance and calmness in the nervous system.

5. Box Breathing (Square Breathing)

Box Breathing involves inhaling, holding the breath, exhaling, and holding the breath again in equal counts. For example, inhale for a count of four, hold for four, exhale for four, and hold for four. This rhythmic pattern promotes relaxation, reduces anxiety, and establishes a sense of control over the breath.

6. 4-7-8 Breathing

Introduced by Dr. Andrew Weil, 4-7-8 Breathing is a simple yet effective technique. Inhale through the nose for a count of four, hold the breath for seven counts, and exhale through pursed lips for eight counts. This pattern induces a sense of calm and can be practiced as needed throughout the day.

7. Sama Vritti (Equal Breathing)

Sama Vritti involves equalizing the duration of inhalation and exhalation. Participants inhale through the nose for a specific count, then exhale for the same count. This balanced breathing technique promotes a calm and centered state, fostering concentration and relaxation.

8. Humming Bee Breath (Bhramari Pranayama):

Humming Bee Breath involves making a humming sound during exhalation.

Participants inhale deeply through the nose and then exhale with a humming sound, prolonging the exhalation. This technique is known for its soothing effect on the nervous system, promoting relaxation and mental clarity.

9. Progressive Relaxation Breathing

Combine deep breathing with Progressive Relaxation by focusing on relaxing different parts of the body sequentially. Inhale deeply, and as you exhale, mentally release tension starting from the toes up to the head. This technique enhances body awareness and contributes to overall relaxation.

10. Guided Visualization Breathing

Incorporate Guided Visualization with breathwork by guiding participants through a mental journey. As they inhale, encourage them to visualize positive images or affirmations. Exhaling, guide them to release any tension or negative thoughts. This integrated approach enhances relaxation and mental clarity.

Encouraging participants to explore and integrate these breathing techniques into their Chair Yoga practice offers a holistic approach to relaxation. As they cultivate a mindful connection with their breath, individuals can tap into the restorative benefits of these practices, fostering a sense of calm, balance, and well-being within the seated context of Chair Yoga.

CHAPTER 4

Chair Yoga Poses for Core Strength

Chair Yoga poses can be adapted to enhance core strength, providing a gentle yet effective way to engage the abdominal muscles and support overall stability. These seated poses target the core while maintaining the accessibility and comfort of practicing with a chair. Integrating these poses into a Chair Yoga routine contributes to building strength in the core muscles, fostering better posture, and supporting overall well-being.

1. Seated Mountain Pose (Tadasana)

While seated on the chair, engage the core by sitting tall, grounding through the feet, and lifting the chest. This foundational pose activates the muscles of the abdomen, promoting core awareness and stability.

2.Seated Twist (Ardha Matsyendrasana)

Incorporate a seated twist by turning the torso gently to one side while holding the back of the chair for support. This engages the obliques and deepens core activation. Alternate between sides to promote balanced strength.

3. Seated Cat-Cow Stretch

Adapt the Cat-Cow Stretch to a seated position by arching and rounding the spine while seated on the chair. This movement engages the core muscles, especially the abdominal muscles, fostering flexibility and strength.

4. Seated Knee-to-Chest Pose

While seated, hug one knee at a time towards the chest. This pose targets the lower abdominal muscles and promotes core engagement. Alternate between legs to provide a balanced workout for the core.

5. Seated Boat Pose Variation

Sit towards the edge of the chair, lean back slightly, and lift the legs off the ground, creating a V-shape with the body. Holding onto the sides of the chair for support, this modified Boat Pose engages the core muscles, especially the lower abdominals.

6. Seated Leg Lifts

Sit with feet flat on the floor, lift one leg at a time straight out in front of you, engaging the abdominal muscles.Repeat with the other leg after lowering it back down.This exercise targets the lower abs and helps build core strength.

7. Seated Side Crunches

While seated, extend one arm overhead and bring the opposite knee towards the elbow in a side crunch motion. This targets the obliques and lateral abdominal muscles. Repeat on both sides to work the entire core.

8. Seated Bicycle Crunches

Place your feet on the floor and take a seat in the chair.Lift one knee towards the chest while simultaneously twisting the torso, bringing the opposite elbow towards the knee. This seated bicycle crunch variation engages both the upper and lower core.

9. Seated Twist with Leg Extension

Combine a seated twist with a leg extension for a dynamic core exercise. Twist the torso to one side while extending the opposite leg. This movement engages the core muscles and promotes balance.

10. Seated Core Activation Breathing

Incorporate intentional breathwork to enhance core engagement. Inhale deeply, engaging the core muscles, and exhale slowly, drawing the navel towards the spine. This controlled breathing while seated activates and strengthens the deep core muscles.

Adding these Chair Yoga poses for core strength to a routine provides a well-rounded approach to enhancing abdominal muscles and overall core stability. Participants can tailor the intensity based on their fitness level while enjoying the accessibility of practicing with a chair. As individuals consistently integrate these poses, they contribute to building a strong and supportive core within the context of Chair Yoga.

Abdominal Exercises

Chair Yoga can be adapted to include effective abdominal exercises, offering a seated and accessible way to strengthen the core muscles. These exercises target various parts of the abdominal region, including the upper and lower abdominals, obliques, and deep core muscles. Incorporating these abdominal exercises into a Chair Yoga routine provides a gentle yet impactful means of improving core strength, stability, and overall well-being.

1. Seated Knee-to-Chest Lifts

While seated, lift one knee at a time towards the chest, engaging the lower abdominal muscles. This exercise strengthens the lower abs and can be performed with a controlled and intentional movement.

2. Seated Leg Raises

Sit at the edge of the chair, keeping the back straight. Lift one or both legs straight out in front of you, engaging the lower abdominal muscles. Lower the legs back down without letting the feet touch the ground. This movement targets the lower abs and hip flexors.

3. Seated Russian Twists

Sit tall on the chair, holding onto the sides for support. Twist the torso to one side, bringing the opposite elbow towards the back of the chair.After circling back to the centre, take a different turn. This exercise engages the obliques and promotes core strength.

4. Seated Bicycle Crunches

While seated, lift one knee towards the chest while simultaneously twisting the torso, bringing the opposite elbow towards the knee. This seated bicycle crunch variation targets the entire core, including the upper and lower abdominals.

5. Seated Side Plank

Hold onto the armrest of the chair and lift your body into a side plank position.From head to heels, maintain a straight body. It works the lateral core muscles as well as the obliques. Switch sides after a few breaths of holding.

6. Seated Toe Touches

Sit with legs extended in front of you. Reach towards your toes, engaging the upper abdominal muscles. This exercise promotes flexibility and strength in the upper abs. Hold for a moment before returning to an upright position.

7. Seated Oblique Crunches

While seated, lean slightly to one side, bringing the elbow towards the hip. This targets the obliques on the side of the torso. Repeat on both sides to work the entire set of oblique muscles.

8. Seated Reverse Crunches

Sit towards the edge of the chair with hands gripping the sides for support. Lift the knees towards the chest, engaging the lower abdominals. Lower the legs back down without letting the feet touch the ground. This exercise targets the lower abs and helps improve core stability.

9. Seated Abdominal Twist with Leg Extension

Sit with feet flat on the floor, twist the torso to one side while extending the opposite leg. This movement engages both the obliques and the lower abdominal muscles. For a well-rounded workout, repeat on the opposite side.

10. Seated Boat Pose

Sit towards the edge of the chair, lean back slightly, and lift both legs off the ground, creating a V-shape with the body.To provide support, hold on to the chair's edges. This modified Boat Pose engages the entire core, including the lower abs and hip flexors.

Incorporating these seated abdominal exercises into a Chair Yoga routine provides a convenient and effective way to strengthen the core muscles. Participants can tailor the intensity based on their fitness level and gradually progress as they build strength and stability in the abdominal region. As with any exercise routine, it's essential to practice with awareness, maintaining proper form and breathing throughout.

Waist-Toning Poses

Waist-toning poses in Chair Yoga focus on engaging the muscles around the waist, including the obliques and the deeper core muscles. These seated postures help to strengthen and tone the abdominal and side body muscles, promoting improved stability and posture. Incorporating waist-toning poses into a Chair Yoga routine provides a gentle and accessible way to target the midsection while enjoying the support of a chair.

1. Seated Side Bend

Sit with a straight spine and feet flat on the ground. Inhale, raise one arm overhead, and exhale while gently bending to the side. This movement targets the obliques and stretches the side body. Repeat on both sides to promote flexibility and tone the waist.

2. Seated Twisting Crunch

While seated, bring one elbow towards the opposite knee, engaging the obliques in a twisting motion. This seated twisting crunch targets the sides of the waist, promoting core strength. Alternate between sides to work both sets of oblique muscles.

3. Seated Side Plank with Leg Lift

Hold onto the armrest of the chair and lift your body into a side plank position. Lift the top leg while keeping the body in a straight line. This combination engages the obliques and tones the waist.Switch sides after a few breaths of holding.

4. Seated Mermaid Pose

Sit with legs extended to the side, one knee bent and the other leg straight. Inhale, raise one arm overhead, and exhale while reaching towards the toes. This pose stretches and tones the side body, targeting the waist muscles. Repeat on both sides.

5. Seated Twisting Boat Pose

Sit towards the edge of the chair, lean back slightly, and lift both legs off the ground. Hold onto the sides of the chair for support and twist the torso to one side. This seated twisting boat pose engages the obliques and deepens core activation, toning the waist. Repeat on both sides.

6. Seated Side Stretch

Sit tall on the chair, inhale, and raise both arms overhead. Exhale while leaning to one side, creating a stretch along the side body. This seated side stretch helps tone the waist and improves flexibility. Repeat on the other side.

7. Seated Waist Rotations

Sit comfortably with a straight spine. Place hands on the waist and gently rotate the torso to one side, then the other. This movement targets the obliques and promotes flexibility in the waist region. Perform the rotations in a controlled manner.

8. Seated Hula Hoop Circles

Imagine drawing circles with the hips while seated on the chair. This rhythmic movement engages the waist muscles and promotes flexibility. Switch directions periodically to work the muscles from different angles.

9. Seated Oblique Crunches

While seated, lean slightly to one side and bring the elbow towards the hip. This seated oblique crunch targets the sides of the waist. Repeat on both sides to work the entire set of oblique muscles.

10. Seated Figure 8s

Draw a figure-eight pattern with the upper body while seated on the chair. This fluid movement engages the waist muscles in a dynamic way, helping to tone and strengthen the core. Perform the figure 8s in a controlled and intentional manner.

Incorporating these waist-toning poses into a Chair Yoga routine provides an effective way to focus on the midsection while respecting the limitations of seated practice. Participants can tailor the intensity based on their fitness level and gradually progress, enjoying the benefits of improved core strength and a toned waistline. As always, it's essential to practice mindfully, paying attention to proper form and breathing throughout the movements.

CHAPTER 5

Chair Yoga for Flexibility

Chair Yoga can be a valuable practice for improving flexibility, making it accessible to individuals with various mobility levels. These seated poses aim to stretch and lengthen muscles, enhance joint mobility, and promote overall flexibility. Integrating Chair Yoga for flexibility into a routine can contribute to increased range of motion, reduced stiffness, and improved joint health.

1. Seated Neck Stretches

Sitting comfortably, gently tilt the head to one side, feeling a stretch along the neck and shoulder. Exchange sides after a few breaths of holding. This increases neck elasticity and relieves tension in the area.

2. Seated Shoulder Rolls

Roll the shoulders forward and backward in a smooth, circular motion while seated. This movement helps relieve tension in the shoulders, promotes flexibility, and enhances range of motion.

3. Seated Side Bend

Sit with a straight spine, inhale, and raise one arm overhead. Exhale while bending gently to the side, feeling a stretch along the torso. This seated side bend improves lateral flexibility and stretches the waist.

4.Seated Forward Bend (Paschimottanasana)

While seated, extend the legs in front and hinge at the hips to reach towards the toes. This seated forward bend stretches the hamstrings and lower back, enhancing flexibility in the spine.

5.Seated Butterfly Pose (Baddha Konasana)

Bring the soles of the feet together and allow the knees to drop outward. Hold the feet and gently press the knees towards the floor. This seated butterfly pose stretches the inner thighs and improves hip flexibility.

6.Seated Wide-Legged Forward Bend

Sit with legs extended wide, inhale, and reach forward toward the center. This stretches the inner thighs, hamstrings, and promotes flexibility in the hips and lower back.

7.Seated Twist (Ardha Matsyendrasana)

While seated, twist the torso gently to one side, using the chair's backrest for support. This seated twist enhances spinal flexibility and releases tension in the back.

8.Seated Ankle-to-Knee Pose (Agnistambhasana)

Cross one ankle over the opposite knee while keeping the back straight. This seated hip opener stretches the outer hips and improves flexibility in the hip joints.

9. Seated Cat-Cow Stretch

Adapt the Cat-Cow Stretch to a seated position by arching and rounding the spine while seated. This movement improves flexibility in the spine and promotes mobility in the back.

10. Seated Leg Stretch with Side Reach

Extend one leg to the side, keeping the other knee bent. Inhale and reach the arm overhead, feeling a stretch along the side body. This seated stretch improves flexibility in the waist and lateral muscles.

11. Seated Twist with Leg Extension

Sit with feet flat on the floor, twist the torso to one side while extending the opposite leg. This combination stretches the spine, waist, and promotes flexibility in the hamstrings.

12. Seated Cow Face Pose Arms

Bring one arm behind the back and the other overhead, attempting to touch the fingers. If fingers don't touch, use a strap or hold onto a cloth. This seated arm stretch enhances shoulder and upper back flexibility.

13. Seated Figure 4 Stretch

Cross one ankle over the opposite knee while keeping the back straight. Gently press down on the raised knee to feel a stretch in the hip and outer thigh. This seated stretch targets the hips and improves flexibility.

14. Seated Hip Opener

Sit towards the edge of the chair, place one ankle on the opposite knee, and gently press down on the raised knee. This seated hip opener stretches the outer hips and enhances hip flexibility.

15. Seated Twisting Wide-Legged Stretch

Sit with legs extended wide, inhale and twist the torso to one side, reaching for the opposite foot. This seated twist stretches the hamstrings and waist, promoting flexibility.

Practicing these Chair Yoga poses regularly can contribute to improved flexibility and overall joint mobility. Remember to breathe deeply, move gently, and listen to your body, allowing for modifications as needed to suit individual comfort levels and physical conditions.

Stretches for Increased Flexibility

Incorporating a variety of stretches into your routine is an excellent way to promote increased flexibility. These stretches target different muscle groups and can be adapted to various fitness levels. Consistent practice of these stretches can contribute to enhanced range of motion, reduced muscle tension, and improved overall flexibility.

1. Neck Stretch

Your ear should be in line with your shoulder as you gently cock your head to one side. Hold for 15-30 seconds, feeling a stretch along the side of your neck. Repeat on the other side.

2. Shoulder Stretch

Bring one arm across your chest, using the opposite hand to gently pull the arm closer. Hold for 15-30 seconds, feeling a stretch in the shoulder and upper back. Switch arms and repeat.

3. Triceps Stretch

Raise one arm overhead and bend the elbow, bringing your hand down your back. Press lightly on the bent elbow with the other hand. Hold for 15-30 seconds, feeling a stretch in the triceps. Repeat on the other side.

4. Chest Opener

Clasp your hands behind your back, straighten your arms, and lift them slightly. Keep your shoulders apart and flex your chest. Hold for

15-30 seconds, feeling a stretch in your chest and shoulders.

5. Cat-Cow Stretch

Start on your hands and knees.Gaze up and raise your head while taking a deep breath (Cow Pose). Exhale, rounding your back and tucking your chin (Cat Pose). Repeat for 1-2 minutes to enhance flexibility in the spine.

6. Seated Forward Bend

Sit with your legs extended in front, hinge at your hips, and reach towards your toes. Hold for 30 seconds, feeling a stretch in your hamstrings and lower back.

7. Butterfly Stretch

Sit with the soles of your feet together, allowing your knees to drop outward. Hold your feet and gently press your knees towards the floor. Hold for 30 seconds, feeling a stretch in your inner thighs.

8. Hip Flexor Stretch

Kneel on one knee, with the other foot in front, forming a 90-degree angle. Find a small stretch in the back leg's hip flexors as you shift your weight forward. Keep each side in place for 30 seconds.

9. Quadriceps Stretch

Stand with your feet hip-width apart. Bend one knee, bringing your heel towards your buttocks, and hold your ankle with your hand. Hold for 15-30 seconds, feeling a stretch in your quadriceps. Repeat on the other leg.

10. Hamstring Stretch

Position your other foot against the inside thigh of the leg that is extended while sitting with one leg extended.Reach towards your toes, feeling a stretch in the hamstring. Hold for 30 seconds on each side.

11. Seated Twist

Sit with your legs extended, cross one foot over the opposite knee, and twist your torso towards the bent knee. Hold for 30 seconds on each side, feeling a stretch in your spine and hips.

12. Ankle Circles

Sit or stand, lift one foot off the ground, and rotate your ankle clockwise, then counterclockwise. Perform ankle circles for 15-30 seconds on each foot to improve ankle flexibility.

13. Wrist Flexor Stretch

Extend your arm in front with palm facing down, use your opposite hand to gently press down on your fingers. Hold for 15-30 seconds, feeling a stretch in your wrist and forearm. Repeat on the other arm.

14. Calf Stretch

Stand facing a wall, place your hands on the wall, and step one foot back with the heel on the ground. Bend the front knee and lean forward, feeling a stretch in the calf. Keep each leg in place for 30 seconds.

15. Seated Yoga Mudra

Sit comfortably, interlace your fingers behind your back, and straighten your arms. Lift your arms slightly, feeling a stretch across your chest and shoulders. Hold for 15-30 seconds.

Remember to perform these stretches gently and gradually, without forcing your body into uncomfortable positions. Incorporate them into your routine regularly, paying attention to your body's feedback, and adjust as needed. Over time, consistent stretching can lead to improved flexibility and a greater sense of overall well-being.

Improving Range of Motion

Improving range of motion involves incorporating targeted exercises and stretches into your routine to enhance the flexibility and mobility of your joints. Whether you're aiming to increase flexibility in specific areas or address overall joint health, consistent practices can contribute to improved range of motion. Here are various approaches and exercises to help enhance your joint mobility:

1. Joint Circles

Perform circular motions with your wrists, elbows, shoulders, hips, knees, and ankles. This dynamic movement helps lubricate the joints, increases synovial fluid production, and gradually improves range of motion.

2. Dynamic Stretching

Include dynamic stretches that involve controlled movements through a full range of motion.Trunk twists, arm circles, and leg swings are a few examples.Dynamic stretching helps warm up the muscles and joints, preparing them for more extensive movement.

3. Foam Rolling

Use a foam roller to release tension in muscles and improve joint mobility. Roll over targeted areas, focusing on muscle groups around the joints. This self-myofascial release technique can enhance flexibility and reduce muscle tightness.

4. Yoga

Engage in regular yoga sessions to promote flexibility and joint mobility. Yoga poses, especially those involving gentle stretches and dynamic movements, contribute to increased range of motion in various joints. Poses like Downward Dog, Warrior series, and Cat-Cow stretches can be particularly beneficial.

5. Resistance Training

Incorporate resistance training exercises that involve a full range of motion. Weightlifting, resistance bands, and bodyweight exercises like squats and lunges can improve joint flexibility when performed with proper technique and form.

6. Static Stretching

Include static stretches after your workout or on rest days. Hold stretches for 15-30 seconds, focusing on major muscle groups and joints. Static stretching helps lengthen muscles, improve flexibility, and gradually enhance range of motion.

7. Pilates

Participate in Pilates, which emphasizes controlled movements and flexibility. Pilates exercises target the core, spine, and various muscle groups, contributing to improved joint mobility and overall flexibility.

8. Swimming

Swimming is a low-impact exercise that engages multiple muscle groups and promotes joint mobility. The resistance of the water supports movement, making it an effective way to enhance flexibility and range of motion.

9. Tai Chi

Practice Tai Chi, an ancient Chinese martial art focused on slow and flowing movements. Tai Chi promotes balance, flexibility, and joint mobility. Regular practice can lead to improved range of motion and increased body awareness.

10. Balancing Exercises

Include balancing exercises that engage the stabilizing muscles around your joints. Single-leg stands, heel-to-toe walks, and balancing on one foot can enhance joint proprioception and stability.

11. Flexibility Training Programs

Follow a structured flexibility training program that addresses specific areas of concern. These programs often include a variety of stretches and exercises tailored to enhance range of motion in targeted joints.

12. Joint Mobility Exercises

Incorporate joint-specific mobility exercises designed to improve the function of specific joints. For example, shoulder circles, hip circles, and ankle circles can be effective in enhancing mobility in those respective areas.

13. Gradual Progression

Focus on gradual progression when introducing new exercises or stretches. Avoid pushing your joints beyond their current limits, and listen to your body's feedback. Consistency and gradual progression are key to long-term improvement in range of motion.

Incorporating a combination of these approaches into your fitness routine can contribute to improved range of motion over time. Consistency, proper form, and mindful progression are essential elements in achieving and maintaining increased joint mobility.

CHAPTER 6

Energizing Chair Yoga Sequences

Energizing Chair Yoga sequences are designed to invigorate the body and mind while being accessible to individuals with varying levels of mobility. These sequences combine gentle movements, breathwork, and stretches to promote energy flow, improve circulation, and enhance overall vitality. Here's a suggested chair yoga sequence to energize your body:

1. Seated Mountain Pose

Sit tall with feet flat on the ground, grounding through your sit bones. Inhale, reaching arms overhead, palms facing each other. Exhale, bringing hands to heart center. Repeat for 5 breaths.

2. Seated Cat-Cow Stretch

Inhale, arching your back and lifting your chest (Cow Pose).Pull your chin in and round your spine as you exhale (Cat Pose). Repeat for 1-2 minutes, syncing breath with movement.

3. Seated Side Stretch

Inhale, lifting one arm overhead, and exhale, bending to the opposite side. Hold for a breath, feeling the stretch along the side body. Repeat on both sides for 5 breaths each.

4. Seated Twist

Stretch your back when you inhale, then release the breath and twist to one side. Grasp the chair's back for assistance. After taking another breath, bring your focus back to the centre. Repeat for 5 breaths on each side.

5. Seated Forward Bend

Inhale, lengthening your spine, and exhale, hinging at your hips to reach towards your toes.

Hold for 5 breaths, feeling a stretch in your hamstrings and lower back.

6. Seated Knee-to-Chest

With both hands, pull one knee towards your chest. Hold for 3 breaths, feeling a gentle stretch in your lower back and hip. Repeat on the other side.

7. Seated Sun Salutation

Incorporate a seated version of Sun Salutation, moving through seated mountain, reaching up, folding forward, and coming back up. Repeat for 5 rounds, syncing breath with movement.

8. Seated Leg Lifts

Sit with feet flat on the ground, lift one leg at a time straight out in front of you. Hold for a breath and lower. Repeat on the other side. Continue for 10 lifts on each leg.

9. Seated Jumping Jacks

While seated, open and close your legs and arms simultaneously, mimicking a seated jumping jack. Engage in this dynamic movement for 1-2 minutes to elevate your heart rate.

10. Seated Breath of Fire

Sit with a straight spine, inhale deeply, and exhale forcefully through your nose. Maintain a rapid and rhythmic breath. Continue for 1-2 minutes, energizing your body with this pranayama technique.

11. Seated Warrior Sequence

Adapt the Warrior sequence to a seated version. Inhale, lifting arms overhead (Warrior 1), exhale, bringing hands to heart center. Inhale, extending one arm forward and the other back (Warrior 2 variation), exhale back to center. Repeat on both sides for 5 cycles.

12. Seated Side Leg Lifts

Sit with one side facing the backrest of the chair. Lift the outer leg out to the side and lower it back down. Repeat for 10 lifts on each side.

13. Seated High Knees

Sit tall and lift your knees towards your chest one at a time, alternating legs in a marching motion. Engage in this movement for 1-2 minutes to boost circulation and energy.

14. Seated Power Breaths

When you raise your arms overhead, take a deep breath through your nose. Exhale forcefully through your mouth, bringing your arms down. Repeat for 1-2 minutes, invigorating your body with powerful breaths.

15. Seated Relaxation

Conclude the sequence with a few minutes of seated relaxation. Close your eyes, focus on your breath, and allow the energizing effects of the sequence to settle.

Modify the intensity and duration of each movement based on your comfort and energy levels. This sequence is adaptable, and you can tailor it to suit your preferences and specific needs. Never ignore your body's signals, and always make the appropriate adjustments.

Invigorating Flow Poses

Invigorating flow poses in Chair Yoga can provide a dynamic and energizing practice while accommodating different levels of mobility. These poses combine movement with breath, creating a flowing sequence that promotes circulation, flexibility, and a sense of vitality. Here's a suggested set of invigorating flow poses that you can integrate into your Chair Yoga practice:

1. Seated Cat-Cow Flow

Inhale, arching your back and lifting your chest (Cow Pose). Take a breath out, tuck your chin, and round your spine to assume the cat pose. Flow between these two poses, synchronizing movement with breath for 1-2 minutes to warm up the spine.

2. Seated Mountain to Forward Fold

Inhale, reaching your arms overhead in Seated Mountain Pose. Exhale, hinge at your hips, and reach forward into a Forward Fold. Inhale back to Seated Mountain. Repeat for 5 rounds, creating a fluid motion.

3. Seated Twist Flow

Release your breath and adopt the cat pose by tucking your chin and rounding your spine.Breathe out to the opposite side and in again towards the centre. Breathe in sync with each twist for a duration of two minutes as you alternate between them.

4. Seated Sun Salutation Flow

Adapt a seated version of Sun Salutation by flowing through Seated Mountain, Forward

Fold, Plank (hands on the sides of the chair, legs extended), and back to Seated Mountain. Repeat for 5 rounds, maintaining a continuous and smooth flow.

5. Seated Warrior Flow

Inhale, lifting your arms overhead (Warrior 1), and exhale, bringing hands to heart center. Inhale, extend one arm forward and the other back (Warrior 2 variation), and exhale back to center. Flow between these variations for 3 minutes, alternating sides.

6. Seated Knee-to-Chest Flow

Inhale, lifting one knee towards your chest, and exhale, extending the leg out. Flow between these movements, alternating legs, for 2 minutes to engage your core and increase circulation.

7. Seated Side Leg Lift Flow

Sit with one side facing the backrest of the chair. Inhale, lift the outer leg to the side, and exhale, lowering it back down. Flow between these movements for 2 minutes on each side, promoting hip mobility and strength.

8. Seated Dynamic Twisting Flow

Stretch your back when you inhale, then release the breath and twist to one side. Inhale back to center and exhale to the other side. Add a dynamic arm movement, reaching the arm behind you as you twist. Flow between sides for 3 minutes.

9. Seated High Knees Flow

Sit tall and lift your knees towards your chest one at a time in a marching motion. Increase the pace, creating a dynamic flow for 2 minutes to boost your heart rate and energize the body.

10. Seated Power Breath Flow

When you raise your arms overhead, take a deep breath through your nose.Exhale forcefully through your mouth, bringing your arms down. Flow between these power breaths

for 2 minutes, invigorating your body with each
cycle.

11. Seated Dynamic Arm Flow

Sit comfortably and flow through dynamic arm
movements, such as arm circles, figure-eights,
and reaching overhead. Explore various arm
movements for 3 minutes to enhance upper
body mobility and energy flow.

12. Seated Leg Extension Flow

Extend one leg at a time, alternating between
legs in a rhythmic motion. Combine this with
dynamic arm movements for 2 minutes,
promoting circulation and engaging the lower
body.

13. Seated Dancing Warrior Flow

Inhale, reaching one arm overhead while lifting
the opposite knee towards your chest. Exhale
back to center and switch sides. Flow between
these dynamic movements for 3 minutes,
adding a dance-like quality to the sequence.

14. Seated Jumping Jacks Flow

While seated, open and close your legs and arms simultaneously in a fluid motion. Engage in this dynamic movement for 2 minutes, bringing an element of cardiovascular exercise into your Chair Yoga practice.

15. Seated Relaxation

Conclude the invigorating flow with a few minutes of seated relaxation. Close your eyes, focus on your breath, and allow the vibrant energy generated during the flow to settle.

Modify the intensity and duration of each movement based on your comfort and energy levels. This invigorating flow sequence is adaptable, and you can tailor it to suit your preferences and specific needs. Never ignore your body's signals, and always make the appropriate adjustments.

Boosting Energy Levels

Boosting energy levels through Chair Yoga involves incorporating dynamic poses, breathwork, and mindful movements to invigorate the body and mind. Here's a set of practices designed to elevate energy:

1. Seated Energizing Breaths

Sit with a straight spine, take a deep inhale through your nose, and exhale forcefully through your mouth. Repeat this energizing breath for 1-2 minutes, focusing on the power of each exhale to release tension and increase alertness.

2. Seated Neck and Shoulder Rolls

Gently roll your shoulders backward and forward, then incorporate neck rolls. This helps release tension in the upper body, promoting relaxation and boosting energy.

3.Seated Spinal Twist with Arm Movement:

Inhale, lengthen your spine, and exhale, twisting to one side. Add a dynamic arm movement, reaching the arm behind you as you twist. Flow between sides for 3 minutes to stimulate the spine and enhance energy flow.

4. Seated Mountain Pose with Arm Circles

Inhale, reaching your arms overhead, and exhale, circling them down and back up. Repeat for 2 minutes, coordinating the movement with your breath to increase circulation and awaken the body.

5.Seated Forward Bend with Dynamic Arm Reach

Inhale, lengthen your spine, and exhale, hinging at your hips to reach towards your toes. Add a dynamic arm reach forward on the inhale and back on the exhale. Flow through this sequence for 3 minutes to stimulate the spine and increase energy.

6. Seated Knee-to-Chest Lifts

Inhale, lift one knee towards your chest, and exhale, lowering it back down. Alternate between legs in a rhythmic motion for 2 minutes, engaging the core and promoting circulation.

7. Seated Dynamic Leg Extensions

Extend one leg at a time, alternating between legs in a rhythmic motion. Incorporate dynamic arm movements to enhance the flow. Engage in this sequence for 3 minutes to activate the lower body and boost energy levels.

8. Seated Sun Salutation

Flow through a seated version of Sun Salutation, moving between Seated Mountain, Forward Fold, Plank (hands on the sides of the chair, legs extended), and back to Seated

Mountain. Repeat for 5 rounds to generate warmth and energy in the body.

9. Seated Warrior Sequence

Inhale, lifting your arms overhead (Warrior 1), and exhale, bringing hands to heart center. Inhale, extend one arm forward and the other back (Warrior 2 variation), and exhale back to center. Flow between these variations for 3 minutes, alternating sides to stimulate the entire body.

10. Seated High Knees with Dynamic Arm Reach

Sit tall and lift your knees towards your chest one at a time, incorporating dynamic arm reaches. Increase the pace for 2 minutes to elevate your heart rate and boost energy levels.

11.Seated Power Breath with Arm Movements

When you raise your arms overhead, take a deep breath through your nose.Exhale forcefully through your mouth, bringing your arms down. Coordinate this power breath with dynamic arm movements for 2 minutes to invigorate your body.

12. Seated Jumping Jacks

While seated, open and close your legs and arms simultaneously in a dynamic motion. Engage in this movement for 2 minutes, introducing a cardiovascular element to increase energy levels.

13. Seated Dancing Warrior Flow

Inhale, reaching one arm overhead while lifting the opposite knee towards your chest. Exhale back to center and switch sides. Flow between these dynamic movements for 3 minutes, bringing a playful and energetic quality to the sequence.

14. Seated Mini Squats

Sit at the edge of the chair, stand up slightly, and lower back down in a controlled motion.

Engage in mini squats for 2 minutes to activate the leg muscles and boost overall energy.

15. Seated Breath of Fire

Sit with a straight spine, inhale deeply, and exhale rapidly through your nose with forceful exhalations. Continue this Breath of Fire for 2 minutes to stimulate the nervous system and increase alertness.

Remember to adapt these practices based on your comfort and energy levels. Always listen to your body, and feel free to modify the movements to suit your individual needs. The goal is to promote a sense of vitality and alertness through the mindful combination of breath and movement.

CHAPTER 7

Mindful Chair Yoga Practices

Mindful Chair Yoga practices involve bringing focused attention to the present moment, combining gentle movements, breath awareness, and meditation while seated on a chair. These practices aim to cultivate mindfulness, reduce stress, and promote a sense of well-being. Here's an explanation of key elements in Mindful Chair Yoga:

1. Mindful Breathing

Begin by sitting comfortably on a chair with your feet flat on the ground. Bring your attention to your breath. Inhale and exhale mindfully, observing the sensation of each breath. Focus on the natural rhythm of your breath, bringing a sense of calmness to your mind.

2. Body Awareness

Scan your body for sensations, starting from your toes and moving up to the crown of your head. Notice any areas of tension or tightness. With each breath, intentionally release tension, allowing your body to relax and be present in the moment.

3. Seated Mountain Pose

Sit with an upright posture, grounding through your sit bones. Imagine yourself as a mountain, stable and rooted. Bring your palms together in front of your heart, fostering a sense of connection between mind and body.

4.Seated Forward Bend with Mindfulness

Inhale, lengthen your spine, and exhale, hinging at your hips to reach forward. Approach the forward bend mindfully, paying attention to the sensation in your hamstrings and lower back. Breathe into any areas of tension, allowing for a gentle stretch.

5. Seated Twists with Awareness

Incorporate gentle seated twists, turning your torso to one side and then the other. As you twist, maintain awareness of the movement, feeling the stretch in your spine and the engagement of your core muscles. Connect each twist with your breath.

6. Mindful Body Scan Meditation

When you close your eyes, focus on various body parts, beginning at your toes and working your way up to the top of your head.Notice any sensations, warmth, or areas of relaxation. This mindful body scan helps deepen your awareness of the present moment.

7. Breath Awareness Meditation

Shift your focus to your breath. Inhale and exhale with intentionality, observing the breath as it enters and leaves your body.Return your attention to the breath gently if it strays. Engage in this breath awareness meditation for a few minutes, cultivating a centered and focused state of mind.

8. Mindful Chair Yoga Flow

Move through gentle and intentional chair yoga poses with full awareness. Whether it's lifting your arms overhead, stretching your legs, or moving in any way, be fully present in the movement. Connect your breath to each pose, creating a seamless flow of mindfulness.

9. Loving-Kindness Meditation

Sit comfortably, close your eyes, and offer kind and loving thoughts to yourself and others. Inhale compassion and exhale any negativity. Extend these wishes for well-being, happiness, and peace to yourself and those around you.

10. Mindful Gratitude Practice

Take a few moments to reflect on aspects of your life that you are grateful for. It could be simple things like the breath you're taking or the support you have. Cultivate a sense of gratitude, allowing it to enhance your overall sense of well-being.

11. Mindful Eating Exercise

If you have a small snack or a piece of fruit, practice mindful eating. Pay attention to the colors, textures, and flavors. Chew slowly, savoring each bite. This practice fosters a connection between mindfulness and daily activities.

12. Mindful Relaxation

Conclude your Mindful Chair Yoga session with a few moments of relaxation. Sit comfortably, focus on your breath, and allow any remaining tension to dissolve. Let your mind and body rest in a state of calm awareness.

Mindful Chair Yoga practices are adaptable and can be tailored to suit individual preferences and needs. The essence lies in bringing a heightened awareness to each moment, fostering a sense of presence and mindfulness in both the body and mind.

Incorporating Meditation

Incorporating meditation into your Chair Yoga practice enhances mindfulness, promotes relaxation, and contributes to an overall sense of well-being. Here's a guide on how to seamlessly integrate meditation into your seated practice:

1. Begin with Mindful Breathing

Start your Chair Yoga session by sitting comfortably with an upright posture. Bring your attention to your breath. Inhale and exhale mindfully, focusing on the sensation of the breath entering and leaving your body. Give yourself a moment to centre yourself with this mindful breathing.

2. Body Scan Meditation

As you settle into your chair, close your eyes and initiate a body scan meditation. Direct your awareness to different parts of your body, starting from your toes and moving up to the crown of your head. Notice any areas of tension or relaxation, bringing a gentle and non-judgmental awareness to each part of your body.

3. Loving-Kindness Meditation

Expand your meditation practice with loving-kindness meditation. Inhale feelings of warmth and compassion, and as you exhale, extend these feelings to yourself and others. Cultivate thoughts of well-being, happiness, and peace.A caring and optimistic outlook is promoted by this practice.

4. Guided Visualization

Incorporate guided visualization into your seated practice. Close your eyes and visualize a peaceful scene, whether it's a calming nature setting or a place that brings you joy. Engage your senses in the visualization, enhancing the overall meditative experience.

5. Mantra Meditation

Choose a simple and soothing mantra, word, or phrase.As you inhale, repeat it aloud to yourself.Allow the mantra to become a focal point for your mind, providing a sense of rhythm and focus. This mantra meditation can help quiet the mind and deepen your state of meditation.

6. Mindful Movement Meditation

Integrate mindfulness into your Chair Yoga movements. As you flow through gentle poses, maintain awareness of each movement and the breath. Connect the physical sensations with your breath, cultivating a moving meditation that enhances flexibility and presence.

7. Breath Awareness Meditation

Focus solely on your breath for a dedicated meditation session. Inhale and exhale naturally, observing each breath without trying to control it. Refocus your attention gently on the breath if your thoughts stray from it. This breath awareness meditation promotes a sense of calm and centeredness.

8.Body Awareness Meditation during Poses

While holding seated yoga poses, practice body awareness meditation. Direct your attention to the sensations in the specific areas of your body engaged in the pose. Notice any warmth, tingling, or stretching sensations, embracing a mindful connection between the body and mind.

9. Mindful Eating Meditation

If you have a small snack or a piece of fruit, practice mindful eating. Engage all your senses as you eat, paying attention to the flavors, textures, and smells. This mindful eating meditation fosters a heightened awareness of the present moment and promotes mindful nourishment.

10. Closing Meditation for Relaxation

Conclude your Chair Yoga practice with a closing meditation for relaxation. Sit comfortably, close your eyes, and guide yourself through a relaxation meditation. Release any remaining tension, and allow your mind and body to rest in a state of calm awareness.

11. Gratitude Meditation

Integrate gratitude meditation into your practice.Think back on the things in your life for which you are happy. Express gratitude for the present moment, your body, and the opportunity to engage in mindful practices. Cultivate a positive and appreciative mindset.

12. Seated Mindful Meditation

Finish your Chair Yoga session with a few minutes of seated mindfulness meditation. Sit with a straight spine, focus on your breath, and allow your mind to settle into a state of quiet awareness. Accept the ease with which you can live in the now.

By incorporating meditation into your Chair Yoga practice, you create a holistic and mindful experience that nurtures both the body and the mind. Feel free to experiment with different meditation techniques to find what resonates best with you, and enjoy the transformative benefits of a combined practice.

Mind-Body Connection in Weight Loss

The mind-body connection plays a crucial role in weight loss, emphasizing the interdependence of mental and physical well-being. By fostering a positive relationship between your mind and body, you can create a more holistic approach to weight loss. Here's an exploration of how the mind-body connection influences weight loss:

1. Mindful Eating

Developing mindfulness around eating involves being fully present and aware during meals. Pay attention to hunger and fullness cues, savor the flavors and textures of your food, and eat without distractions. This mindful approach helps regulate portion sizes, prevent overeating, and enhances the overall eating experience.

2. Emotional Eating Awareness

Understanding the emotional triggers behind eating habits is crucial. Emotional eating, which can be prompted by stress, boredom, or other emotions, can lead to weight gain.By addressing the root causes of these triggers and substituting healthier coping mechanisms, awareness of these triggers can help you lessen your dependency on food for emotional comfort.

3. Stress Management

Hormonal abnormalities, especially elevated cortisol levels, can result from long-term stress and could potentially cause weight gain.Incorporating stress management techniques such as meditation, yoga, or deep breathing exercises can help regulate stress hormones and support weight loss efforts.

4. Positive Body Image

Cultivating a positive body image is vital for long-term weight management. Embrace your body with love and acceptance, focusing on the aspects you appreciate. This positive mindset fosters a healthier relationship with your body, motivating you to make sustainable lifestyle choices rather than engaging in restrictive diets or excessive exercise.

5. Goal Setting and Visualization

It's critical to set attainable and realistic weight loss goals.Visualize your success and imagine the positive changes in your life as you work towards these goals. Visualization can enhance motivation, boost confidence, and create a more positive mindset conducive to successful weight loss.

6. Intuitive Movement

Listen to your body's signals and engage in physical activities that bring joy and fulfillment. Adopting an intuitive movement approach allows you to connect with your body's needs, promoting consistent exercise that aligns with your preferences and lifestyle.

7. Body-Mind Exercises

Practices like yoga, Pilates, and tai chi promote the integration of body and mind. These exercises focus on controlled movements, breath awareness, and mindfulness, fostering a deeper connection with your body while improving strength, flexibility, and overall well-being.

8. Self-Compassion

Practicing self-compassion is integral to a healthy mind-body connection. Be kind to yourself during the weight loss journey, acknowledging that setbacks and challenges are a natural part of the process. This compassionate approach helps build resilience and prevents negative self-talk that can hinder progress.

9. Sleep Quality

Establishing healthy sleep patterns is crucial for weight management.A disturbed hormonal balance brought on by sleep deprivation can intensify cravings and hunger.Prioritize adequate and quality sleep to support overall well-being and weight loss efforts.

10. Holistic Nutrition

Adopting a holistic approach to nutrition involves choosing nutrient-dense foods that nourish both the body and mind. Make sure your diet is well-balanced and full of whole foods, such as fruits, vegetables, lean meats, and whole grains.Proper nutrition supports physical health while positively impacting mental clarity and mood.

11.Mindfulness-Based Weight Loss Programs

Explore mindfulness-based weight loss programs that integrate meditation, mindful eating practices, and psychological support. These programs address both the physical and emotional aspects of weight loss, providing a comprehensive approach to achieving and maintaining a healthy weight.

12. Behavior Change Techniques

Incorporate behavior change techniques that align with your mindset and preferences. Whether it's setting small, achievable goals, using positive affirmations, or tracking progress, these techniques can enhance motivation and create a sustainable path toward weight loss.

13. Professional Support

Consider seeking support from healthcare professionals, including registered dietitians, psychologists, or counselors specializing in weight management. Professional guidance can provide personalized strategies, address underlying emotional factors, and offer a structured approach to achieving weight loss goals.

14. Mindful Hydration

Stay mindful of hydration as it influences various bodily functions, including metabolism. Drinking water mindfully, especially before meals, can contribute to a sense of fullness, supporting portion control and overall weight management.

15. Journaling and Reflection

Maintain a journal to track your thoughts, feelings, and behaviors related to weight loss. Regular reflection allows you to identify patterns, celebrate achievements, and gain insights into the mind-body connection, fostering self-awareness and growth.

By acknowledging and nurturing the mind-body connection in weight loss, you create a foundation for sustainable and positive changes. Embracing a holistic approach that considers both physical and mental well-being enhances the likelihood of successful and lasting weight management.

CHAPTER 8

Chair Yoga for Stress Reduction

Chair Yoga can be a valuable tool for stress reduction, offering accessible and gentle practices that promote relaxation and calmness. Here's an exploration of Chair Yoga techniques tailored for stress relief:

1. Seated Breath Awareness

Start by sitting comfortably on a chair with your feet flat on the ground.Focus on your breathing while you close your eyes. Inhale deeply through your nose, feeling your chest and abdomen rise, and exhale slowly through your mouth. Focus on the sensations of each breath, allowing your mind to center on the present moment.

2. Neck and Shoulder Release

Your ear should be facing your shoulder as you gently cock your head to one side.Remain in this position for several breaths, allowing your neck's side to feel stretched.Repeat on the other side. For your shoulders, inhale as you lift them toward your ears, and exhale as you release them down. Repeat these movements to release tension in the neck and shoulders.

3. Seated Cat-Cow Stretch

Sit with a straight spine, place your hands on your knees, and inhale as you arch your back (Cow Pose). Lift your chin up to your chest in the cat pose as you release the breath. Flow between these two movements with your breath, creating a gentle seated version of the traditional Cat-Cow stretch.

4. Seated Forward Bend

Inhale, lengthen your spine, and exhale as you hinge at your hips, reaching forward toward your feet. Allow your hands to rest on your shins or the floor. Hold the stretch for a few breaths, feeling a release in your lower back and hamstrings.

5. Seated Twist

Inhale to lengthen your spine, and exhale as you twist gently to one side, placing one hand on the opposite knee and the other behind you for support. Twist again on the opposite side, holding it for a few breaths. Twisting poses are effective for releasing tension in the spine and promoting relaxation.

6. Seated Heart Opener

Sit near the edge of the chair, place your hands on the backrest, and gently open your chest by lifting your heart towards the ceiling. Take slow and deep breaths, feeling the expansion across your chest. This pose counteracts the hunched posture often associated with stress.

7. Mindful Arm Movements

Inhale as you lift your arms overhead, and exhale as you bring them down. Focus on the fluidity of the movement and synchronize it with your breath. This mindful arm movement helps release tension and promotes a sense of calm.

8. Seated Meditation

Take a comfortable seat, close your eyes, and focus within. Focus on your breath or use a guided meditation for stress reduction. Allow any intrusive thoughts to pass without judgment, and gently bring your focus back to your breath.

9. Legs-Up-the-Chair Pose

Lie on your back and extend your legs up against the seat of a chair.Use a cushion if necessary to support your lower back.This gentle inversion helps promote relaxation, improve circulation, and reduce stress.

10. Guided Relaxation

Finish your Chair Yoga session with a guided relaxation.Release tension by concentrating on every area of your body. Visualize a calm and peaceful place. Allow yourself to fully relax, integrating the benefits of the practice into your mind and body.

11. Chair Yoga Nidra

Explore a guided Chair Yoga Nidra session for deep relaxation. This guided meditation involves systematic relaxation and can be particularly effective in reducing stress and promoting a sense of inner calm.

12. Mindful Breathing Techniques

Incorporate specific mindful breathing techniques such as diaphragmatic breathing, box breathing, or alternate nostril breathing. These techniques activate the parasympathetic nervous system, inducing a relaxation response and reducing stress.

13. Hand and Finger Relaxation

Bring your attention to your hands and fingers. Gently stretch and release each finger, then rotate your wrists. This simple practice can help release tension in the hands, which often carry stress.

14. Seated Hip Opener

Sit with your feet flat on the ground and open your knees to the sides.Grasp the chair's sides for assistance. This pose gently opens the hips, releasing stored tension and promoting relaxation.

15. Mindful Movement Sequences

Create short mindful movement sequences by combining several Chair Yoga poses in a fluid and intentional manner. Sync the movements with your breath, allowing for a seamless and calming practice that reduces stress.

Regularly incorporating these Chair Yoga techniques into your routine can contribute to stress reduction and promote a greater sense of calm and well-being. Remember to listen to your body and adapt the practices to suit your comfort and needs.

Relaxation Techniques

Relaxation techniques encompass various practices aimed at reducing stress, promoting calmness, and fostering a sense of well-being. These techniques are designed to evoke the body's relaxation response, counteracting the effects of stress on both the mind and body. Here's an explanation of some commonly used relaxation techniques:

1.Deep Breathing (Diaphragmatic Breathing)

Explanation: Deep breathing involves inhaling slowly through the nose, allowing the diaphragm to fully expand, and exhaling through the mouth. This technique promotes relaxation by activating the body's parasympathetic nervous system, leading to decreased heart rate and blood pressure.

2.Progressive Muscle Relaxation (PMR)

Reason: Progressive muscle relaxation (PMR) entails systematically tensing and relaxing various muscle groups. Starting from the toes and moving upward, this technique helps release physical tension and promotes a deep sense of relaxation throughout the body.

3.Guided Imagery and Visualization

Explanation: Guided imagery encourages the use of vivid mental images to create a sense of relaxation. This technique often involves imagining a peaceful and serene place, engaging the senses to enhance the overall experience and reduce stress.

4.Mindfulness Meditation

Explanation: Mindfulness meditation involves bringing one's attention to the present moment without judgment. This can be achieved through focused breathing, body scans, or simply observing thoughts and sensations. Mindfulness helps cultivate a non-reactive awareness, reducing stress and promoting mental clarity.

5.Autogenic Training

Explanation: Autogenic training involves self-suggestion and imagery to induce a state of relaxation. Practitioners repeat a series of phrases related to warmth and heaviness, promoting a sense of calmness and reducing stress.

6.Yoga and Tai Chi

Explanation: These mind-body practices combine gentle movements, breath control, and meditation. Yoga and Tai Chi are effective for reducing stress, improving flexibility, and promoting a sense of balance and well-being.

7.Biofeedback

Explanation: Biofeedback involves monitoring physiological functions such as heart rate, muscle tension, or skin temperature. By providing real-time feedback, individuals can learn to consciously control these bodily responses, leading to relaxation and stress reduction.

8.Aromatherapy

Explanation: Aromatherapy utilizes essential oils to promote relaxation and reduce stress. Inhaling or applying essential oils can have calming effects on the nervous system. Scents like lavender, chamomile, and eucalyptus are commonly used for relaxation.

9.Massage Therapy

Explanation: Massage involves manipulating soft tissues to relieve tension and promote relaxation. The physical touch and pressure applied during a massage stimulate the release of endorphins, reducing stress and enhancing overall well-being.

10. Hypnosis

Explanation: Hypnosis involves guided relaxation and focused attention to induce a trance-like state. In this state, individuals may be more receptive to suggestions for behavioral changes or stress reduction. It can be performed by a trained practitioner or through self-hypnosis techniques.

11. Breath Control Techniques (Pranayama)

Explanation: Pranayama, a component of yoga, encompasses various breath control techniques. Techniques like alternate nostril breathing or rhythmic breathing can positively influence the autonomic nervous system, promoting relaxation.

12. Tai Chi

Explanation: Tai Chi is a gentle martial art characterized by slow and flowing movements. It incorporates deep breathing and meditation, fostering relaxation, balance, and flexibility. Regular practice can contribute to stress reduction.

13.Self-Compassion Practices

Explanation: Cultivating self-compassion involves treating oneself with kindness and understanding. Practices may include positive affirmations, acknowledging one's feelings without judgment, and fostering a nurturing and supportive inner dialogue.

14.Grounding Techniques

Explanation: Grounding techniques involve bringing attention to the present moment by connecting with the physical environment. This may include feeling the texture of an object, focusing on the breath, or engaging in mindful walking to reduce stress and anxiety.

15.Journaling and Relaxation Exercises

Explanation: Journaling about thoughts and feelings, as well as engaging in relaxation exercises, such as progressive muscle relaxation or guided meditation, can provide an outlet for self-expression and contribute to stress reduction.

It's important to note that the effectiveness of relaxation techniques can vary among individuals. Exploring different methods and finding what resonates best with personal preferences is key to establishing a regular relaxation practice. Additionally, incorporating these techniques into a consistent routine can enhance their long-term benefits for overall well-being.

Stress and its Impact on Weight

Stress can have a significant impact on weight, influencing both behaviors and physiological processes that contribute to weight gain. Here's an in-depth exploration of how stress affects weight and contributes to changes in eating habits and metabolism:

1. Hormonal Responses

Cortisol Release: The hormone linked to the body's "fight or flight" reaction is released in response to stress. Chronic stress can lead to elevated cortisol levels, which may contribute to increased abdominal fat storage. This type of fat distribution is linked to a higher risk of metabolic issues.

2. Appetite Regulation

Ghrelin and Leptin Imbalance: Stress can disrupt the balance of hunger and satiety hormones, such as ghrelin and leptin. Elevated cortisol levels may increase appetite, particularly for high-calorie, comfort foods.Overindulgence and eventual weight gain may result from this mismatch.

3. Emotional Eating

Stress-Induced Cravings: Many individuals turn to food as a coping mechanism during times of stress. The desire for comfort foods, often high in sugar and fat, can be driven by the brain's response to stress.Increased calorie intake and weight gain can be caused by emotional eating.

4. Metabolic Changes

Insulin Resistance: Chronic stress is associated with insulin resistance, where the body's cells become less responsive to insulin. This condition can lead to elevated blood sugar levels and an increased risk of developing type 2 diabetes. Insulin resistance is also linked to weight gain, especially around the abdominal area.

5. Sleep Disruption

Impact on Sleep Quality: Stress can disrupt sleep patterns, leading to insufficient or poor-quality sleep. Sleep deprivation affects the regulation of hunger hormones, increasing ghrelin and decreasing leptin, which can contribute to overeating and weight gain.

6. Coping Mechanisms

Unhealthy Coping Habits: Individuals experiencing chronic stress may resort to unhealthy coping mechanisms, such as overeating, consuming excessive alcohol, or adopting a sedentary lifestyle. These behaviors can contribute to weight gain and negatively impact overall health.

7. Physical Inactivity

Reduced Exercise Motivation: Chronic stress may reduce motivation for physical activity. Lack of exercise can contribute to weight gain and exacerbate the physiological effects of stress on the body.

8. Digestive Issues

Gut-Brain Connection: The gut-brain axis plays a role in stress-related digestive issues. Stress can lead to changes in gut microbiota and increased permeability of the intestinal lining. These alterations may influence weight regulation and metabolic health.

9. Genetic Factors

Interaction with Genetic Predispositions: Genetic factors can influence an individual's susceptibility to stress and its impact on weight. Some individuals may be more prone to stress-induced changes in appetite, metabolism, and weight regulation.

10. Long-Term Health Consequences

Chronic Health Conditions: Prolonged exposure to stress and its associated impact on weight can contribute to the development of chronic health conditions, including obesity, cardiovascular disease, and metabolic syndrome.

11. Vicious Cycle

Stress-Weight Gain Cycle: Stress can create a vicious cycle where weight gain and its associated health consequences become sources of additional stress. Breaking this cycle often requires addressing both the psychological aspects of stress and adopting healthier lifestyle habits.

12. Mind-Body Connection

Psychological Impact: Stress has a profound psychological impact, influencing mood, motivation, and self-control. Individuals under chronic stress may find it challenging to adhere to healthy eating patterns and maintain a physically active lifestyle.

Understanding the intricate relationship between stress and weight is crucial for implementing effective strategies for weight management. Combining stress-reduction techniques, such as mindfulness, meditation, and adequate sleep, with healthy lifestyle choices can contribute to overall well-being and support weight-related goals. Seeking professional guidance, including consultation

with healthcare providers or nutritionists, can
also be beneficial for addressing stress-related
weight concerns.

CHAPTER 9

Nutritional Tips for Weight Loss

Effective weight loss involves a combination of a balanced and nutrient-dense diet, along with healthy lifestyle habits. Here are nutritional tips to support weight loss:

1. Calorie Control

Create a Caloric Deficit: To lose weight, consume fewer calories than your body expends. A moderate calorie deficit, typically 500 calories per day, can lead to gradual and sustainable weight loss.

2. Balanced Macronutrients

Include Protein, Healthy Fats, and Carbohydrates: Ensure each meal includes a balance of protein, healthy fats, and carbohydrates. Protein helps maintain muscle mass, while healthy fats and complex carbohydrates provide sustained energy.

3. Portion Control

Be Mindful of Portions: Pay attention to portion sizes to avoid overeating. You can help control portion sizes by using smaller bowls, plates, and utensils and by paying attention to your body's signals of fullness and hunger.

4. Proper Hydration

Remain Hydrated Throughout the Day by Drinking Enough Water. Gluttony can occasionally be confused with a dehydration crisis. Drinking water before meals may also help control appetite.

5. Whole Foods Emphasis

Prioritize Whole, Unprocessed Foods: Choose whole, nutrient-dense foods such as fruits, vegetables, whole grains, lean proteins, and healthy fats. These foods provide essential vitamins, minerals, and fiber while helping control overall calorie intake.

6. Limit Added Sugars

Reduce Sugar Intake: Minimize the consumption of foods and beverages high in added sugars. Opt for natural sweeteners or sources of sweetness from fruits.

7. Fiber-Rich Foods

Increase Fiber Intake: Include high-fiber foods like fruits, vegetables, whole grains, and legumes in your diet.Fibre encourages satiety, which lowers total calorie intake and helps you feel full for longer periods.

8. Time of Meals

Consume Frequently: Create a regular schedule for meals and snacks to help you maintain a consistent eating pattern. Not eating can result in overeating later in the day, so try not to skip meals.

9. Eatables High in Nutrients

Select Nutrient-Dense Snacks: Select nutrient-dense snacks like a handful of nuts, Greek yoghurt with berries, or raw veggies with hummus. Energy levels are maintained in between meals thanks to this.

10. Mindful Eating

Practice Mindful Eating: Pay attention to your eating experience by savoring each bite, chewing thoroughly, and avoiding distractions. Mindful eating promotes awareness of hunger and fullness cues.

11. Meal Prep

Plan and Prepare Meals: Plan your meals in advance, and prepare healthy options to avoid relying on convenience or fast food. This allows you to have control over ingredients and portion sizes.

12. Healthy Cooking Methods

Opt for Healthier Cooking Techniques:
Choose cooking methods such as grilling,
steaming, baking, or sautéing instead of frying.
These methods help retain nutritional value
without excess added fats.

13. Probiotic-Rich Foods

Include Probiotics: Incorporate foods rich
in probiotics, like yogurt, kefir, or fermented
vegetables. Probiotics support gut health,
which is linked to overall well-being and weight
management.

14. Stay Consistent

Consistency is Key: Make sustainable
changes to your eating habits rather than
opting for restrictive diets. Attaining and
sustaining weight loss requires consistency
over an extended period.

Remember, successful weight loss involves a
holistic approach that combines healthy eating
with regular physical activity and other lifestyle

factors. It's essential to adopt sustainable habits that align with your individual preferences and needs.

Healthy Eating Habits

Healthy eating habits are essential for maintaining overall well-being, supporting optimal physical and mental health, and preventing various chronic diseases. Here's an in-depth exploration of key healthy eating habits:

1. Balanced Diet

Include a Variety of Foods: Consume a well-rounded diet that includes a variety of fruits, vegetables, whole grains, lean proteins, and healthy fats.You'll be guaranteed to get a wide range of vital nutrients this way.

2. Portion Control

Be Mindful of Portions: Pay attention to portion sizes to avoid overeating. Use smaller plates and be conscious of hunger and fullness cues to maintain a healthy balance.

3. Regular Meals

Establish Regular Eating Times: Aim for regular meals and snacks throughout the day. This helps stabilize blood sugar levels and prevents excessive hunger, reducing the likelihood of unhealthy food choices.

4. Hydration

Drink Plenty of Water: Stay adequately hydrated by drinking water throughout the day. In addition to helping with digestion and appetite control, water supports a number of biological processes.

5. Limit Processed Foods

Minimize Processed and Ultra-Processed Foods: Reduce the intake of foods high in added sugars, refined carbohydrates, and artificial additives. Focus on whole, minimally processed options.

6. Moderation

Enjoy Treats in Moderation: While prioritizing nutrient-dense foods, allow yourself occasional treats. Enjoying indulgent foods in moderation can help maintain a balanced approach to eating.

7. Mindful Eating

Eat with Awareness: Practice mindful eating by paying attention to each bite, savoring flavors, and recognizing hunger and fullness cues. Avoid distractions like screens during meals.

8. Slow Eating

Chew Food Slowly: Chew your food thoroughly. Eating slowly allows your body to recognize when you are satisfied, preventing overeating.

9. Meal Preparation

Meal Preparation and Planning: When feasible, prepare your meals at home using a prearranged menu. Making better decisions is facilitated and you have control over the ingredients.

10. Incorporate Whole Grains

Select Whole Grains: Make sure to choose whole grains such as oats, brown rice, quinoa, and whole wheat. Essential nutrients and fibre are found in whole grains, which support healthy digestive function.

11. Lean Proteins

List the Sources of Lean Proteins. Fish, poultry, beans, lentils, tofu, and low-fat dairy are examples of lean protein sources. Protein helps maintain the health of muscles, promotes fullness, and assists in controlling body weight.

12. Healthy Fats

Accept Healthy Fats: Consume foods high in avocados, nuts, seeds, and olive oil, among other sources of healthy fats. These fats are beneficial for heart health and contribute to overall well-being.

13. Limit Added Sugars

Reduce Added Sugar Intake: Minimize the consumption of sugary beverages, desserts, and processed snacks. Choose naturally sweet options like fruits when seeking sweetness.

14. Diverse Colorful Plate

Prioritize Colorful Foods: Aim for a diverse and colorful plate. Different colors in fruits and vegetables signify various nutrients, antioxidants, and health benefits.

15. Listen to Your Body

Respond to Hunger and Fullness: Pay attention to your body's hunger and fullness signals.When hunger strikes, eat, and when satisfaction strikes, stop.

16. Culinary Herbs and Spices

Enhance Flavor with Herbs and Spices:
Use herbs and spices to flavor your dishes
instead of relying on excessive salt or
high-calorie sauces. This adds variety to your
meals without compromising health.

17. Read Food Labels

Understand Food Labels: When
purchasing packaged foods, read labels to
understand the nutritional content. Pay
attention to serving sizes, sugar content, and
overall nutrient composition.

18. Limit Processed Meats

Moderate Processed Meat Consumption:
Limit intake of processed meats like bacon,
sausages, and deli meats, which may be high in
salt and additives.

19. Social Eating

Be Mindful in Social Settings: Practice
healthy eating habits when dining out or
attending social events. Make conscious

choices and balance indulgences with nutritious options.

By adopting these healthy eating habits, you can foster a positive relationship with food, support your body's nutritional needs, and contribute to long-term well-being. Remember that small, sustainable changes over time can lead to significant improvements in your overall health and nutritional habits.

Nutrient-Rich Foods

Nutrient-rich foods are those that provide a high concentration of essential vitamins, minerals, antioxidants, and other beneficial compounds relative to their calorie content. Including these foods in your diet helps ensure you meet your nutritional needs while promoting overall health. Here's an in-depth exploration of various nutrient-rich foods across different food groups:

1. Leafy Greens

> ➤ **Examples:** Spinach, kale, Swiss chard, collard greens.

> ➤ **Nutrient Highlights:** Rich in vitamins A, C, K, and folate, as well as minerals like iron and calcium. These greens also contain antioxidants and fiber.

2. Berries

> ➤ **Examples:** Blueberries, strawberries, raspberries, blackberries.

> ➤ **Nutrient Highlights:** Packed with antioxidants, vitamins (C and K), and fiber. Berries also provide natural sweetness without added sugars.

3. Cruciferous Vegetables

> ➤ **Examples:** Broccoli, cauliflower, Brussels sprouts, cabbage.

> ➤ **Nutrient Highlights:** High in vitamins C and K, fiber, and various

phytochemicals with potential health benefits, including anti-cancer properties.

4. Nuts and Seeds

- ➢ **Examples:** Almonds, walnuts, chia seeds, flaxseeds.
- ➢ **Nutrient Highlights:** Good sources of healthy fats, including omega-3 fatty acids. Nuts and seeds also provide protein, fiber, vitamins, and minerals.

5. Fatty Fish

- ➢ **Examples:** Salmon, mackerel, trout, sardines.
- ➢ **Nutrient Highlights:** Rich in omega-3 fatty acids, which are beneficial for heart health. Fatty fish also provide high-quality protein, vitamins D and B12, and minerals like selenium.

6. Whole Grains

> **Examples:** Quinoa, brown rice, oats, barley.

> **Nutrient Highlights:** Excellent sources of complex carbohydrates, fiber, vitamins (B vitamins), and minerals (iron, magnesium). Whole grains contribute to sustained energy and digestive health.

7. Legumes

> **Examples:** Chickpeas, lentils, black beans, kidney beans.

> **Nutrient Highlights:** High in plant-based protein, fiber, and an array of vitamins and minerals, including folate, iron, and potassium.

8. Greek Yogurt

> **Nutrient Highlights:** Rich in protein, calcium, probiotics (beneficial for gut

health), and various vitamins. Opt for plain, unsweetened Greek yogurt for lower added sugars.

9. Colorful Vegetables

➢ **Examples:** Bell peppers, carrots, sweet potatoes, tomatoes.

➢ **Nutrient Highlights:** Vibrant vegetables provide a spectrum of vitamins, such as A and C, as well as antioxidants. They contribute to immune function and overall health.

10. Eggs

➢ **Nutrient Highlights:** Excellent source of high-quality protein, vitamins (B2, B12, D), and essential minerals (iron, zinc). Eggs also contain choline, important for brain health.

11. Lean Poultry

> **Examples:** Chicken breast, turkey.

> **Nutrient Highlights:** High-quality protein, B vitamins (especially niacin and B6), and minerals like phosphorus and selenium.

12. Dairy (or Dairy Alternatives)

> **Examples:** Milk, cheese, fortified plant-based milk (almond, soy).

> **Nutrient Highlights:** Rich in calcium, vitamin D, protein, and other essential nutrients.Make healthier choices by selecting low-fat or non-fat options.

13. Colorful Fruits

> **Examples:** Oranges, bananas, apples, mangoes.

> **Nutrient Highlights:** Fruits provide a variety of vitamins (C, potassium, folate)

and antioxidants. A natural supply of dietary fibre is also provided by them.

14. Avocado

- ➢ **Nutrient Highlights:** Packed with heart-healthy monounsaturated fats, avocados also provide fiber, vitamins (K, C, E), and minerals (potassium).

15. Tomatoes

- ➢ **Nutrient Highlights:** Rich in vitamins (C, K), antioxidants like lycopene (linked to heart health), and potassium. Tomatoes can be consumed fresh or in various processed forms like sauces.

16. Bell Peppers

- ➢ **Nutrient Highlights:** High in vitamins (C, A), fiber, and various antioxidants. Bell peppers come in different colors, each offering unique nutritional benefits.

17. Dark Chocolate (in Moderation)

> **Nutrient Highlights:** Contains antioxidants, especially flavonoids. Dark chocolate may have heart-protective effects and can contribute to mood improvement.

18. Green Tea

> **Nutrient Highlights:** Rich in antioxidants, particularly catechins. Green tea may have various health benefits, including supporting metabolism and reducing the risk of certain diseases.

19. Seaweed (Nori)

> **Nutrient Highlights:** An excellent source of iodine, essential for thyroid health. Seaweed also provides vitamins (A, C, B vitamins) and minerals (calcium, iron).

20. Mushrooms

> **Nutrient Highlights:** Low in calories and rich in vitamins (D, B vitamins) and minerals (selenium, copper). Some mushrooms may have immune-boosting properties.

Incorporating a diverse array of nutrient-rich foods into your diet ensures that you receive a broad spectrum of essential nutrients, promoting overall health and well-being. Remember to focus on variety, moderation, and balanced meals to support your nutritional needs.

BONUS

30-Day Chair Yoga Challenge

30-Day Chair Yoga Challenge can be a great way to introduce individuals to a series of poses that promote flexibility, strength, and relaxation. Here's an outline with explanations for each pose:

Week 1: Introduction to Chair Yoga

Day 1: Seated Mountain Pose

Explanation: Sit tall with feet flat on the ground. Place hands on thighs, lengthen the spine, and breathe deeply. This pose establishes a foundation for proper seated posture.

Day 2: Seated Forward Bend

Explanation: Sit at the edge of the chair, hinge at the hips, and reach toward the floor. This pose stretches the spine, hamstrings, and promotes flexibility in the back.

Day 3: Seated Twist

Explanation: Sit tall, twist the torso gently to one side, and use the chair's back for support. Repeat on the other side. This pose enhances spinal flexibility and aids digestion.

Day 4: Neck and Shoulder Rolls

Explanation: Sit comfortably, roll the shoulders back and forth, and gently move the neck in circular motions. This helps release tension in the neck and shoulders.

Day 5: Seated Cat-Cow Stretch

Explanation: Sit with a straight spine, place hands on knees, and arch the back (Cow Pose), then round the back (Cat Pose). Repeat to improve flexibility and mobility in the spine.

Day 6: Wrist and Ankle Rotations

Explanation: Rotate wrists and ankles in both directions to improve joint mobility. This is especially beneficial for those spending extended periods sitting.

Day 7: Seated Butterfly Stretch

Explanation: Sit tall, bring soles of feet together, and gently press knees toward the floor. The hips and inner thighs are stretched in this pose.

Week 2: Building Strength and Stability

Day 8: Seated Leg Lifts

Explanation: Sit at the edge of the chair, lift one leg at a time, engaging the core. This strengthens the abdominal muscles and improves leg strength.

Day 9: Seated Knee Extension

Explanation: Sit tall, extend one leg at a time, and hold. This pose targets the quadriceps and helps improve knee flexibility.

Day 10: Seated Side Leg Lifts

Explanation: Sit tall, lift one leg to the side, and lower it with control. This strengthens the outer thighs and hips.

Day 11: Seated Figure Four Stretch

Explanation: Cross one ankle over the opposite knee, gently press the knee down. This stretches the outer hip and glutes.

Day 12: Seated Boat Pose

Explanation: Sit tall, lift legs off the ground, balancing on the sit bones. Engage the core. This pose strengthens the abdominal muscles.

Day 13: Seated Warrior Pose

Explanation: Sit tall, extend one leg back with toes pointing, engage the core.Pose for improved balance and leg strength.

Day 14: Seated High Lunge

Explanation: Sit at the edge of the chair, step one foot back into a lunge position. This strengthens the legs and works on stability.

Week 3: Flexibility and Relaxation

Day 15: Seated Forward Fold with Twist

Explanation: Sit tall, fold forward, and add a gentle twist. This stretch targets the spine, hamstrings, and improves rotational flexibility.

Day 16: Seated Pigeon Pose

Explanation: Sit tall, cross one ankle over the opposite knee, gently press down. This stretches the outer hip and glutes.

Day 17: Seated Child's Pose

Explanation: Sit back on the chair, reach arms forward, and lower the chest. This pose provides a gentle stretch for the back and shoulders.

Day 18: Seated Side Stretch

Explanation: Sit tall, reach one arm overhead, and gently bend to the side. This stretch targets the side body and promotes lateral flexibility.

Day 19: Seated Tree Pose

Explanation: Sit tall, place one foot on the inner thigh of the opposite leg. This pose improves balance and stretches the inner thighs.

Day 20: Seated Eagle Arms

Explanation: Sit tall, cross one arm over the other, and bring palms together. This stretch targets the shoulders and upper back.

Day 21: Seated Restorative Pose

Explanation: Sit comfortably, close the eyes, and focus on deep breathing. This pose promotes relaxation and mindfulness.

Week 4: Putting It All Together

Day 22: Seated Sun Salutation

Explanation: Combine seated mountain pose, forward bend, and other poses in a flowing sequence. This builds heat, flexibility, and engages the entire body.

Day 23: Seated Flow Sequence

Explanation: Move through a series of seated poses with fluid transitions. This sequence enhances flexibility and brings awareness to breath and movement.

Day 24: Seated Balance Poses

Explanation: Explore seated balance poses, such as lifting one foot off the ground or balancing on the toes. This challenges stability and strengthens core muscles.

Day 25: Seated Meditation

Explanation: Sit comfortably, focus on the breath, and cultivate a sense of calm. This meditation practice enhances mindfulness and relaxation.

Day 26: Seated Heart-Opener

Explanation: Sit at the edge of the chair, place hands on the backrest, and gently arch the back. This pose opens the chest and promotes an uplifted posture.

Day 27: Seated Twisting Flow

Explanation: Combine seated twists with flowing movements. This sequence enhances spinal mobility and engages the core.

Day 28: Seated Savasana

Explanation: Sit comfortably, close the eyes, and relax. This final pose allows for reflection and deep relaxation.

Day 29: Seated Gratitude Meditation

Explanation: Reflect on gratitude while seated comfortably. This meditation fosters a positive mindset and a sense of appreciation.

Day 30: Seated Celebration Pose

Explanation: Celebrate the completion of the challenge with a seated posture of choice. This can be a moment to express gratitude and acknowledge progress.

Remember to encourage participants to listen to their bodies, modify poses as needed, and approach the challenge with a sense of curiosity and self-compassion.

Tracking progress and results

Tracking progress and results is a crucial aspect of any wellness journey, including a 30-day Chair Yoga Challenge. This process not only provides motivation but also helps individuals assess the impact of their efforts. Here's an expanded guide on tracking progress and results:

1. Establish Clear Goals

Explanation: Clearly define specific and realistic goals for the Chair Yoga Challenge. These goals could include improved flexibility, reduced stress, enhanced balance, or increased mindfulness. Having specific objectives provides a clear focus for tracking progress.

2. Create a Daily Journal

Explanation: Maintain a daily journal to record thoughts, feelings, and experiences related to each yoga session. Document any changes in mood, energy levels, or physical sensations. This can serve as a personal reflection and help identify patterns over time.

3. Take Before and After Photos

Explanation: Capture photos at the beginning and end of the challenge to visually track changes in posture, flexibility, and overall well-being. Visual documentation provides a tangible way to observe progress.

4. Keep a Practice Log

Explanation: Maintain a log of the specific poses practiced each day, duration, and any modifications made. This log helps individuals track consistency, identify favorite poses, and note areas for improvement.

5. Use a Rating System

Explanation: Implement a daily rating system to assess the perceived difficulty or comfort level of each yoga session. This subjective feedback allows participants to track their evolving experience throughout the challenge.

6. Measure Physical Changes

Explanation: Take physical measurements before and after the challenge to monitor changes in flexibility, strength, or balance. This objective data can provide concrete evidence of progress.

7. Track Emotional Well-Being

Explanation: Incorporate a mood or emotional well-being tracker into the progress monitoring process. Note changes in stress levels, mood, and overall mental health throughout the challenge.

8. Assess Sleep Quality

Explanation: Keep track of sleep patterns and quality during the challenge. Improved sleep can be a positive outcome of regular chair yoga practice, contributing to overall well-being.

9. Monitor Stress Levels

Explanation: Use stress assessment tools or personal reflection to monitor stress levels. Regular chair yoga can have a significant impact on stress reduction, and tracking stress levels provides insights into its effectiveness.

10. Document Challenges and Breakthroughs

Explanation: Record any challenges faced during the Chair Yoga Challenge and note breakthrough moments. Documenting obstacles and successes helps individuals learn and adjust their approach.

11. Weekly Check-Ins

Explanation: Schedule weekly check-ins to review progress and make any necessary adjustments to goals or routines. This regular assessment provides an opportunity for reflection and refinement.

12. Celebrate Milestones

Explanation: Acknowledge and celebrate milestones achieved during the challenge. Whether it's mastering a challenging pose or consistently practicing, recognizing achievements fosters motivation.

13. Gather Feedback

Explanation: Seek feedback from participants about their experiences and perceived benefits. This information can inform future practices and help refine the Chair Yoga Challenge for others.

14. Reflect on Mindfulness

Explanation: Reflect on the mindfulness aspects of the challenge. Note any changes in awareness, focus, or the ability to stay present during yoga sessions. Mindfulness gains are valuable outcomes.

15. Post-Challenge Reflection

Explanation: Conduct a comprehensive post-challenge reflection. Assess overall progress, identify areas for continued growth, and set new goals or intentions for the future. Encouraging participants to actively engage in tracking their progress enhances their commitment to the Chair Yoga Challenge. The combination of subjective and objective measures allows for a holistic understanding of the impact of chair yoga on physical and mental well-being.

CONCLUSION

"Chair Yoga for Women to Lose Weight" serves as a transformative journey, empowering every reader to embrace wellness through the gentle yet potent practice of yoga. As you close this book, remember that the strength to change lies within, and the support of a chair becomes a symbol of resilience. Each pose, each breath, and each moment of mindfulness contributes to a profound shift not just in physicality but in the very essence of your being.

This 30-day challenge is not merely a guide; it is an invitation to rediscover your body's wisdom and nurture a harmonious connection between mind, body, and spirit. Your progress, whether visible or felt within, is a testament to your commitment and capacity for transformation.

As you carry the lessons of chair yoga into your daily life, may the practice become a sanctuary a refuge where self-love, strength, and balance thrive. Embrace the journey ahead with gratitude, and let this book be a companion on your path to lasting well-being. Remember, every breath is an opportunity for renewal, and every pose is a step toward the vibrant, empowered version of yourself.

May the wisdom shared within these pages inspire a lifelong commitment to self-care, mindful movement, and the enduring belief that you possess the power to sculpt a healthier, happier existence. Your body is a vessel of strength, your mind a reservoir of resilience, and your spirit an unwavering source of vitality. With this, go forth, embark on your journey, and may each day be a celebration of the remarkable journey that is your life. Namaste.